T0153038

POWER
VEGAN

POWER VEGAN

Plant-Fueled Nutrition for Maximum Health and Fitness

REA FREY

SURREY
BOOKS

AN AGATE IMPRINT

CHICAGO

Copyright © 2013 by Rea Frey

All rights reserved. No part of this book may be reproduced or transmitted in any form or by any means, electronic or mechanical, including photocopying, recording, or by any information storage and retrieval system, without express written permission from the publisher.

All photographs copyright © 2013 by Nikki McFadden Photography

Design by Brandtner Design

Printed in the United States of America.

Library of Congress Cataloging-in-Publication Data

Frey, Rea.
 Power vegan : plant-fueled nutrition for maximum health and fitness / by Rea Frey.
    pages cm
 Includes bibliographical references and index.
 Summary: "A guide to developing a plant-based diet for improved nutrition, fitness, and health.
 Includes recipes and exercises"-- Provided by publisher.
 ISBN 978-1-57284-141-3 (pbk.) -- ISBN 978-1-57284-722-4 (ebook)
 1. Vegan cooking. 2. Vegetarianism. I. Title.
 TX837.F725 2013
 641.5'636--dc23

2013008710

10 9 8 7 6 5 4 3 2 1

Surrey is an imprint of Agate Publishing. Agate books are available in bulk at discount prices.
For more information, go to agatepublishing.com.

To all the plants who give their lives to make mine better—thank you.

CONTENTS

ACKNOWLEDGMENTS

Thank you to the wonderful team at Agate, who allowed me to write the book I've always wanted to write. Your steadfast advice and encouragement are rare in this business.

Thanks to Heather Crosby of YumUniverse for supplying endless dinner recipes when I was too tired to come up with my own (and for contributing a few to the Power Vegan Recipes chapter as well). Thank you to Brendan Brazier, who continues to shed light on how easy and successful a vegan life can be, and has inspired me in numerous ways, both on the page and off. Thanks to Jonathan Safran Foer for his enlightening book *Eating Animals*, which prompted me to dive back in to a vegan life. Thanks to Nikki McFadden, who stayed up all night, rode a disgusting bus, and shot the exercise photos on no sleep. You are a photography ninja.

And thanks to my husband, Alex, who chops, cooks, folds, cleans, loves, smiles, parents, impersonates, laughs, and provides the best companionship one could ask for. Thank you for the humor, the friendship, the love, and the loyalty. Thank you for being my first reader, my sounding board, my exception. Thank you for it all.

PREFACE

Wednesday, May 30, 2012
3:51 a.m.

I look in the mirror set in front of me. My face is crimson. I've been pushing for two hours. Somehow, after much protest, I've ended up flat on my
back, with my knees in the air. I've been going at this for exactly 52 hours.
Those tiny bits of banana, blackstrap molasses, and coconut water my
doula kept sneaking me have long since worn off. I am ravished.

"It's a cone head," Dr. Lin says. "A really big cone head." After my
daughter's head is out, it takes five more pushes to get her body to escape
mine. I have never been so exhausted. Fifty-two hours. Fifty-two hours
of contractions. Fifty-two hours with minimal food and fluids. Fifty-two
hours without sleep. Fifty-two hours of relaxation, fear, agony, and bliss.
Fifty-two hours to change my life.

The doctor hands her to me. There is a collective gasp as I clutch her
to my chest, unsure what to feel, so exhausted I can barely keep my eyes
open. There are no tears, only wonder.

I feel her head, sprinkled with hair, resting against my hospital gown.
I see her face, crumpled and serene. But she is not crying. She is slightly
blue. She's been stuck for far too long, and rather than bonding with me as
I'd planned, she is whisked off to get things moving. The cord is clamped.
I watch them take her from me, and I hear myself ask that dreaded ques-
tion: "Is she okay?"

The silence is deafening. But she is okay. She is better than okay. She is
perfect. Already, I know that she is a fighter. We have waged the ultimate

war together. We have had one of the longest journeys to meet each other, and from here on out, nothing will ever be as hard as our voyage to get her here.

After this, I can do anything.

They finally bring her to me, freshly swaddled. I touch her face. I clutch her long fingers with the beautifully shaped fingernails. I look at my husband, Alex, who has been by my side the entire time. I smile at my doula and at my mother, who has been watching from the corner of the room. I stare at my daughter, rolling the unfamiliar word around in my mouth.

"Holy shit," I say. "I did it. Now when can I eat?"

I have always been a voracious eater. To say I once had a "healthy" appetite would be a severe understatement. What I had was the mindset of an overeater. As I ate breakfast, I daydreamed about my midmorning snack, my lunch, and what my parents would make for dinner. What I would have after dinner. What I could eat *between* dinner and that after-dinner snack.

Sometimes, if I was in a bad mood, I would think about the delectable treats that awaited me (an entire Sara Lee pie, a tray of fish sticks, a whole box of macaroni and cheese!) and I would instantly brighten. It went hand in hand with thinking about watching a brand-new episode of *90210* or dressing up and watching *Flash Gordon* with my brother in our tiny living room—these were the things I lived for as a child.

As soon as my mother finished putting away the groceries, I would demolish everything: five boxes of cereal, a tin of blueberry muffins with butter, cinnamon toast, a complete carton of eggs, a huge jug of orange juice, an entire box of chicken tenders. You name it, I ate it. Perhaps this was due in part to the fact that I was an avid gymnast, hurtling my body through the air. I wore my bumps and bruises proudly, shouting to anyone who would listen: "I'm an athlete."

As a young adult, I gave up meat and fell prey to numerous fad diets. Though I wasn't overweight, I was weight obsessed and in dire need of good, quality calories from high-nutrient foods to support my intense physical exertion. Instead of feeding my body healthy food, I would eat entire sleeves of fat-free saltines slathered with fat-free cream cheese; large bags of baked Lays with Olestra; or fat-free, sugar-free chocolate pudding.

I would limit calories, fat, and sugar, pumping my body full of chemicals and depriving it of proper nutrition. As I grew older and the demands on my body grew heavier with sports, I began to educate myself.

I became a group exercise instructor at 17 and a personal trainer at 18. I got certified in weight management, sports nutrition, fitness nutrition, and plant-based nutrition. Over the years, I've taught people what it means to pay attention to their bodies and not a diet book. I've helped them identify the implications of their everyday choices and become more aware of what they are eating and why. I've helped supply recipes and resources. I've gotten them off their scales and in tune with how their bodies are feeling, not just what they look like.

After dealing with a couple of treacherous health scares of my own (a daunting foray into brain surgery and a botched knee surgery), I began to abhor traditional medicine due to its tendency to address the symptom and not the actual problem. So I started to look into the power of food to help me heal. I examined my life and all the stressors in it and began to make connections with what I ate, who I kept company with, and how I felt. I started asking questions: What does it mean to eat for health and not out of convenience? What does it mean to listen to my body instead of the FDA? Since the FDA was a business, wasn't it important to do my homework on what it actually researched and supported, as well as what it left out? What about advertisers? Do they care about my health or just selling products? How can I tune all this out and bring vitality into my body in other ways?

On my journey, I have learned a lot. I am still learning and will continue to educate myself, regardless of how many seminars I attend, research I complete, or certifications I obtain.

And while there are numerous ways to eat (just Google "diets" and scroll through the results), the ideas for health that this book offers are simple. Whether your goal is improved stamina for workouts, weight loss, or a cure for persistent ailments, you can reach it through the following principles, which I have put to work in my career and my own life:

- Ignore diets. If diets worked, there would only be one.
- Pay attention to how you feel after you eat. Your body indicates what it likes, what gives it energy, what it's allergic to, and what makes it feel terrible. We are programmed to know the foods we should be eating if we simply pay attention.
- Eat what you like. By pinpointing the foods you can't live without, you don't have to diet to achieve health. You can learn to eat better versions of them and make yourself feel better in the process. (There are some caveats to this, of course. If all you love are french fries and pizza, there are still ways to enjoy them—albeit in smaller doses and with better ingredients.)
- Eat whole foods. Whole foods come from the ground (and don't have a heartbeat). This doesn't mean that you have to be a vegetarian or that meat is awful—only that the bulk of your diet should come from fresh produce, healthy seeds, nuts, grains, and legumes.

Not a day goes by that I don't feel the effects of the food I eat. It's an awareness that I carry with me, like the bumpy scar on my scalp and the shifts in my body since becoming a mother.

And while I never thought I would become a parent, I know I have a very big job ahead of me in teaching my daughter what nutrition means. I can control the food my daughter eats now because my body produces it, but I know there will be a time when I cannot. Someday she will be cast out into the world, where the norm is to eat fast food and birthday cake. Will she be the weirdo who refuses candy because she knows how it affects her body? Isn't it a kid's right to be hopped up on sugar from time to time? Will she be able to understand how our bodies aren't meant to eat all these processed foods, and see how they are literally killing our nation? Or will she blend into the crowd?

Just as I will teach my daughter the virtue of good, clean food and continue to promote our idea of living a balanced, healthy life, ultimately the choice is hers. I don't own her. I will trust her enough to make her own decisions. I will not know more about her nature than she does, nor will I know what foods will make her feel best. The work will be up to her. I will just provide the tools to help her get there.

While there's so much we cannot control in this world, there is a vital component to life that is completely in our control: what we eat. Eating is the only thing we do numerous times per day, every day, for our entire lives. Every food choice we make has an effect: on how that food is processed in our bodies, how it makes us feel, how it is assimilated, how it leaves our bodies, or how it collects in and damages them—later leading to clogged arteries or causing obesity and disease.

Somewhere along the way we have gotten off track. We have gotten away from paying attention to how the foods we eat make us feel and, more importantly, what they are doing to us.

Altering my thought process to what I call "power eating" has changed my life—and quite possibly saved it.

I invite you to do the same, a single principle at a time.

INTRODUCTION: LET'S EAT

"Let food be thy medicine and medicine be thy food." —HIPPOCRATES

What does it mean to be a Power Vegan eater (and no, this does not mean ramming copious amounts of food down your throat for a competitive eating contest)?

The term "power" is associated with strength. We know the power of politics and our government. We know the power of bodybuilders and the power of nature. But we so rarely think about the power of the food we eat, and how it affects us both inside and out.

From the time we are born, we are introduced to food. Perhaps it begins with our mother's breast milk ("liquid gold," as it's often called, because it is made specifically for our bodies and can protect us from any harmful bacteria or viruses). Our diets quickly unravel to less healthy fare from there, as traditions are passed down, convenience foods are sought, and we instantly develop a taste for all things sugary, quick, and indulgent.

We're taught that for strong bones we need dairy. To build muscle, we need protein, and that protein needs to come from an animal. If we want to be "strong," we eat a solid American diet of meat, potatoes, and side dishes that come from a box.

But why not rearrange the American diet to center around vegetables, fruits, grains, seeds, and healthy legumes, the benefits of which have been proven time and time again? What would that food pyramid look like, and what would it mean for our health?

The fact is that we can bring real power into our bodies with the food that we eat. This book will show you how to lay down a solid foundation for the bulk of your diet. If you can do the groundwork, everything is more manageable, regardless of whether you're stressed, you eat out often, or you have cravings. By making the majority of your diet plant based (and yes, that means you can still throw in organic, lean meats and dairy when you want to), you can set yourself up for permanent success and improved health, even if you fall off the wagon from time to time.

Power Vegan eating is a way of eating that can work for you, even if you've been raised on fast food and microwave dinners. You can turn it around simply and effectively by shifting your focus to more greens, produce, seeds, nuts, grains, legumes, and other natural foods that don't take a lot of preparation or come from a package.

The truth? Collectively, Americans are unhealthy. The American Heart Association reported in 2012 that, among Americans 20 years and older, 149.3 million are overweight. Of these, 75 million are obese.[1] We have extremely high death rates from non-communicable diseases (NCDs), such as stroke, diabetes, cancer, and premature heart disease. For the 36 million deaths reported from NCDs in 2008, the World Health Organization reported that 80 percent of the contributing risk factors were preventable.[2]

To many, these statistics aren't a surprise. What is a surprise is that you can prevent common diseases that often cause premature death by changing what you eat. You can alleviate almost any physical ailment, allergy, or mental and emotional complaint by shifting what you put into your mouth.

When you constantly tax your body with sugar, processed foods, and chemicals, you are prohibiting your body from doing what it's meant to do. Instead of giving you energy, it struggles to break down and get rid of this waste. Over time, you will suffer from physical ailments, nutritional stress, pain, and eventually illness and disease.

Power Vegan focuses on foods that give you energy and vitality. Foods that come from the ground; foods that haven't been overly processed or poured into toxic cans or plastic bags. Foods that are portable, tasty, and uncomplicated and have been proven time and time again to boost health and nutrition. Foods that are alive, meaning that they haven't been cooked at high temperatures, drowned in butter, or ground to virtually unrecognizable versions of themselves. Foods that are simple and wholly intact; foods in their natural state.

You can incorporate these foods into your diet however you see fit. Slowly, you can start to educate yourself on what's right for your body (not your partner's or your kids' or your best friend's) and figure out how you feel and what's the best "recipe" for your level of health. There is no diet to power eating.

Regardless of whether you are looking to shift your way of eating for life, for health, for a specific ailment, for your age, for fitness, or because you want to eat like an athlete, *Power Vegan* will help you attain your goals to reach optimal health. It will provide the tools to get healthy with sound information about foods for daily life. It's about fitting in the healthy concepts you need while ditching the rest of the extreme health noise out there.

No diets. No complicated recipes. Just powerful foods for a powerful life.

The Keys to Your Health

You know the drill. Go to a restaurant. Order what looks good. Salivate. Have bread. Have olive oil. Have a drink. Have a steak. Eat. Eat a lot. Eat way too much. Fall into a food coma for the rest of the night. Render yourself useless in front of the television. Get up and do the same thing tomorrow. Gain five pounds. Gain ten pounds. Become sluggish. Blame the restaurants. Buy bigger clothing. Go on a diet. Get cranky. Stop going to restaurants. Get on the wagon. Fall off the wagon. Repeat. Repeat. Repeat.

Our internal health is the catalyst for most external issues. No matter how healthy or unhealthy you feel, we all suffer from certain ailments that are a product of the choices we make when it comes to exercise, eating, and our lifestyles.

We are not born liking pizza. We are not born liking cookies. These are the foods we grow up with in America. We forget how amazing a piece of fruit can taste, or how wonderful a bowl of fresh vegetables can be. We forget that our bodies are made to move, that we have a brilliant resiliency within us, and that if we just acknowledge the choices we make and stop running ourselves into the ground, we can make our lives and our bodies extraordinary.

When it comes to being healthy, the definitions are vast and often superficial. In our society, health is usually defined exclusively by what you look like on the outside. As long as we're eating low-fat, low-carb fare (often laden with chemicals), then we're healthy, right? Wrong. Look at the ingredients on everything you eat and even put in your body. (Tip: If you can't pronounce it, don't eat it!)

We all want that "quick fix" to get healthy. We want big results in the shortest amount of time with the least amount of effort. The reality? There is no magic pill that will make you healthy. Regardless of everything you've read, getting healthy involves more than just trying a new diet or exercise plan. It's the correlation between how you live, what you eat, and how you move your body. They are all connected. And once you find the perfect recipe for your body, you can live a healthier, more balanced life—no medicine or expensive programs required.

It's time to make your lifestyle choices work for you and not against you. We're taught that to have the bodies and the health we want is difficult. In fact, it's the complete opposite. We were intended to live healthy lives, but we have so much junk in our bodies and our minds that we often feel disconnected from our lives, our jobs, our friends, our bodies, and our partners. As a result, we become unhealthy in ways that range from nagging little aches and pains to major exhaustion, stress, and weight gain. We'd rather give up than make an effort to do what it takes to change.

But there is a way to eradicate all of these issues using simple, plant-based foods (and no, you don't have to be a vegan or even a vegetarian to benefit from this way of eating). There is a way to pinpoint the cause of your ailments, just by paying attention to how you feel. There is a way to alter your diet, your movement patterns, and possibly the stressors in your life with no complicated recipes or steps. And every single day, you can have clear, healthy skin, feel radiant and strong, be at the weight you desire, and move through the world the way you always intended to.

Most of us don't know what it's like to exist at optimal levels of health. We think our joints naturally hurt with age, our metabolisms slow; that we need deodorant because we are supposed to smell, that we get exhausted after giant pasta dinners, and we need caffeine to stay awake. It's simply our way of life. We do little to question or change it. It's just easier to accept things the way they are instead of challenging the system.

If we do want to reach optimal levels of health, we assume it will involve weird food concoctions, years of detoxing, and a general unhappy way of living that revolves around deprivation and isolation.

This is not the case.

Power Vegan delivers the only solution you will ever need. The key? Individuality. No two bodies are the same, so how can we expect to find one way of eating that works for everyone? Today there are so many different ways of eating, endless exercises to try, and numerous ways to organize your personal life and your love life. In a word: overwhelming. But, there's good news. Our bodies are incredibly smart. If we listen, they can tell us exactly what we should and shouldn't be eating.

By paying attention to your likes and dislikes, you can meet your own personal health quota each and every day. Hate to cook? Find recipes that are easy and take no more than 20 minutes to make (most of the recipes in Chapter 13 fall into this category). If you constantly crave sweets, find easy, healthy alternatives that are satisfying and not just low-fat, chemical-laden versions of the original. Most important? Know what you're not willing to do. If you hate going to the grocery store, then perhaps you need a delivery service or personal grocery shopper. If you don't like to chop veggies, buy them pre-cut. Don't like salads? Don't eat salads. Hate raw foods? Don't eat raw foods.

Healthy is about finding what you enjoy and what you're willing to do to get there. It's not about eating perfect or looking perfect. It's about knowing. If you have the knowledge for your individual physique, you can make more educated choices about what you put into your body and how it affects you. You become more in tune with how you feel, period.

This way of eating and paying attention is sustainable. There's no 30-day approach. It's a daily approach. You get up, you make smarter choices today, and you do the same thing tomorrow. You are building a lifestyle shift, not a five-day or five-week shift. You are the one who's responsible for your own success. It's about making choices that work for you and your life, in all capacities.

SELF-ASSESSMENT: EMOTIONAL HEALTH

Just as we are connected to one another, our bodies are connected to our minds. So much about being healthy goes beyond the physical. The first step is to look at all aspects of your life. If you are unhappy in any area, take a few minutes to self-assess and figure out why. For those questions to which you answer yes, you'll find solutions in the self-evaluation section below. (You will find similar self-assessments throughout this book that focus on different aspects of eating and health.)

1. Am I unhappy in my relationship?

2. Do I feel drained when I spend time with certain friends?

3. Am I miserable in my job?

4. Am I stressed about money?

EVALUATE YOUR ANSWERS

If you find that you are unhappy in your personal relationships, assess whether the issues are big or small. For instance, if your romantic partner doesn't respect you, that's a big issue. If a friend is constantly late to scheduled meetups, that's a smaller issue. It's important to determine what's fixable and what's not, and to look at your own baggage, as opposed to someone else's. Make sure you are accepting your partner and friends for who they are instead of who you might want them to be.

If you find instead that most of your emotional stress comes from job or money woes, you are definitely not alone. Perhaps you hate your job and count down the hours until you can leave every day. If so, it may be time to take the road less traveled and figure out what you might be able to do differently in order to be happier and more productive. Can you live with less? Then perhaps you can branch out and follow that artistic dream. If you can't survive without a steady paycheck, have a heart-to-heart with your boss about salary or expectations.

If money is your biggest stressor, take a hard look at your spending, which can reveal hidden culprits that could be draining your bank account (and your mental health). Go through bills and bank statements to see where the bulk of your spending happens. Concoct tangible ways to earn more and spend less.

Improving the emotional factors in your life can enhance health, slash stress, and free up time and attention to focus on food and exercise. The important thing is to tend to your needs—all of your needs—because you can eat all the plants in the world, hit the gym seven days a week, and still not reach your goals if you are unhealthy in other areas of your life. Look at getting healthy as a progressive, daily challenge.

Tips for Using This Book

There are numerous ways to use this book. You can skip to the chapters you are most interested in and use them for your specific needs and purposes, you can read from start to finish, you can go directly to the self-assessments, or you can dive into the recipe or workout sections. This book is here to help guide you and bring you new ways of thinking, eating, and being that work for you, not against you.

IF YOU'RE VEGAN

If you're vegan, chances are you can use a bit of a reminder about how to get the vitamins and minerals you need, how best to avoid certain nutrient deficiencies, and how foods affect your body and performance. As you read, think about where your diet can use improvement, how you feel, what vitamins and minerals you might be lacking, and how you can bring more energy into your everyday life with simple recipes, fresh ingredients, and attention to how your body feels.

SELF-ASSESSMENT: WHAT KIND OF VEGAN ARE YOU?

Ask yourself what kind of vegan you are by using the following questions, and read on for how to evaluate your answers.

1. *Do I like to eat fake meats and cheeses to mimic an American diet?*

2. *Do I eat a lot of processed foods and carb-heavy meals?*

3. *Do I eat mostly raw foods but skimp on proteins?*

4. *Do I eat the same things every day?*

EVALUATE YOUR ANSWERS

If you gravitate toward processed foods, it's time to look at the ingredients lists. Veggie meats often have long lists of processed ingredients and are laden with sodium. Figure out what you love about these foods: is it the texture, the taste, or both? If you love burgers, perhaps try making your own black bean burgers from scratch, or fill up on healthy legumes and start to shift your taste buds so you don't always reach for the fake stuff. If you can't give up your fake hot dogs, limit them to just a few times per week and fill up on unprocessed foods whenever possible.

Eating raw foods is wonderful, as all plants contain protein. However, if you only eat vegetables and never reach for legumes or other plant-based proteins, you could be missing out on vital nutrients imperative for building and repairing lean muscle (see Chapter 3). On the other hand, if you always buy the same fruits, vegetables, and grains at the store, step outside the box. Instead of eating kale every day, opt for romaine, mustard greens, Swiss chard, or escarole. Love strawberries? Reach for raspberries, blueberries, or blackberries instead. Addicted to almond butter? Try sunflower seed butter, cashew butter, or even pumpkin seed butter. Check out the list of power foods in Chapter 1. Aim for new ingredients each week to see how your body responds.

Regardless of how you eat, *Power Vegan* can show you that you don't need fake meat to be a vegan; that fresh foods can translate into satisfying, comforting fare; and that you can get a variety of vitamins and minerals by eating what's in season and frequenting your market to whip up easy dishes. Focus on flavor—it makes all the difference when it comes to satiating your appetite.

|||||||||||||||||||||||||||||||||||||||||||||||||||||||||||||||||||||||||||||||||||||||||||||||||||||||||||||||||||||||||||||||||||||||||||||||||||

IF YOU'RE NOT VEGAN

Perhaps you have zero interest in giving up steak or chicken or cheese. That's completely fine. If you feel great eating these foods, continue to eat them. You can use this book to improve your health, help aid your pre- and post-exercise nutrition, find new recipes suitable for the entire family, boost your workouts, and better understand the nutrients you need, regardless of your diet.

You can learn to pinpoint certain allergic reactions that may be brought on by food and figure out how to eradicate them with exercise, lifestyle changes, and simple foods that are cheaper, healthier, and all-around better for you (see page 164). Pay attention to the quizzes in this book and assess and reassess how you feel after every single meal. You can reach optimum levels of health and fitness by following my guidelines and taking an individual approach.

And, if you are interested in plant-based eating, start small. One day per week, have a meatless day and see how you feel. Then you can start adding in plant-based days from there.

Bottom Line

Power Vegan isn't about what you cut from your diet, it's about what you *add*. Use this book to figure out what needs to be tweaked in your diet and your life. Focus on factors in your job, your relationship, your finances, and your personal life that could be affecting how you eat or how you feel about food in general.

Pinpointing the triggers in your life can help eliminate them once and for all. Just take it a single step at a time.

CHAPTER 1

Power Vegan Principles

"If you don't take care of your body, where are you going to live?"

—UNKNOWN

"How can I explain this so that it makes sense?"

I stared at my husband, whose six-pack abs contracted as he stirred oatmeal.

"I'm not sure," he said. "I wish there were just three rules you could give people to show them how easy getting healthy really is."

"But people don't like rules."

He looked at me, that devastating smile altering the features of his face. "Well, people don't like rules, but they like results. And these aren't rules in the traditional sense. They're easy. I've followed them, your clients have followed them, and everyone has success. Voilà." He lifted the spoon, a few hot pieces of oats splattering our hardwood floor. Neruda, our puppy, was there in an instant, scalding her tongue to devour them.

I studied Alex, this specimen who was my best work. As a certified nutrition specialist and sports-specific trainer, I had worked with him to devise a way of eating and moving that worked with and for his body.

"I never thought I'd have abs. I thought I would always be a fat tub of goo."

"You were never a fat tub of goo."

"Yes, I was."

"No, you weren't. But it's hilarious how now you can't stop staring at yourself in the mirror."

He loaded the spoon again, a new mound of oats ready to launch my way.

"It's your fault. You did this to me. I blame you entirely."

When we'd met, he'd been 50 pounds heavier. He played rugby. He could bench press 420 pounds. He'd been an athlete most of his life (and had the massive legs to prove it), but he was only eating three times per day. He had no meal structure. He would often eat two entrées at a time, and work out around the clock. He ate out most meals. He was tired and sore and not sleeping well. While not fat, he definitely had a layer that wasn't muscle, and though he had a good knowledge base of what he should and shouldn't be eating, he wasn't eating for energy or ingesting the types of foods his body needed for such powerful activities.

We related to each other instantly. We both ate copious amounts of food and often curtailed that intake with increased exercise. But after reading *Eating Animals*, *The China Study*, and *Thrive*, each of which takes a different approach to the benefits of a plant-based lifestyle, I was contemplating returning to plant-based eating. It wasn't that I thought eating meat was terrible, but I felt better without it. I began gravitating toward clients who were vegetarians or vegans and started comparison studies on those who ate a plant-based diet versus a traditional American diet. The results were astounding, especially for athletes. Those who ate plant-based meals recovered more quickly, had a lower resting heart rate, a lower body fat percentage, lower cholesterol, and increased strength and endurance.

For Alex, however, I used my sports nutrition background to shift his meals to seven per day, leaving meat and dairy in. Within a month, 20 pounds fell off—just by eating more.

While he lost weight but maintained lean muscle, we began frequenting restaurants most nights of the week. I saw the scale creep up and my own clothes grow tighter. I began to feel lethargic. Having been a gymnast, a weightlifter, and a boxer most of my life, I didn't like what I saw or felt. I had always been a compulsive eater—often thinking about my next meal before I finished my current one—but exercise usually made up for any excess food intake.

As I became more informed about what food was actually doing to my body and how exhausting digestion really is, I began to think about what was happening internally—not just what I looked like.

What happens when we eat, exactly? While digestion begins in our mouths, we rarely think beyond swallowing (and later eliminating). Once food enters, chewing and salivary enzymes begin to break it down. From the mouth, food moves on to the esophagus and makes its way to the stomach. The esophagus is so strong, you can eat or drink while upside down.

Food then enters the stomach and gets doused by gastric acid and other acids, known as chyme. Food flows into the small intestine, where bile and other enzymes help further break it down. It then passes to the large intestine, where water and electrolytes are removed. Food travels up toward the ascending colon and then back down to the descending colon before turning into waste and being excreted.

Total time from mouth to excretion? Though this depends on the nature of the food and the individual's body, according to the Mayo Clinic and Dr. Michael F. Picco, digestion can take anywhere from 40 to 50 hours from start to finish.[3]

If you're constantly eating, your body is constantly working to digest that food, instead of supplying you with energy for other activities. Eating nutrient-dense, energy-efficient foods can help give the body a break. As compared to a piece of meat, a handful of seeds (which packs just as much protein) is a lot easier and kinder for the gut to break down. Not only that, but if we're constantly cramming our mouths with what we don't need, we put constant strain on our bodies, which can lead to a host of health problems over time.

Once I had a better idea of what was happening inside my body, I began to ponder all the other products I was using in my home and wondered if they could be having an effect on my health as well. I ransacked my house and looked at every item I owned. Why did I buy this brand of soap, that kind of yogurt, or this specific type of perfume? What were advertisers telling me to buy, and why was I complying? What was I putting in my body and on my body? And could it be affecting how I felt?

I began to simplify, swapping chemical-laden cleaners for vinegar and water, and swapping natural makeup for the popular brands and gentle baby washes with no harsh ingredients instead of harsh soaps with fragrances.

Armed with extensive research and a dose of healthy inspiration, I decided I definitely wanted to venture back to the realm of a plant-based life. I had gone vegetarian before, beginning when I was 13 and continuing for approximately 13 years. But now I was hesitant about actually giving up meat, dairy, and eggs, so I broached the subject with Alex. In my earlier years as a vegetarian, I thought eating black beans and broccoli would suffice. I knew better now. If I went back down that road, I wanted to cover all the nutrition bases I had learned about: protein; healthy fats; good grains, such as buckwheat, quinoa, millet, wild rice, teff, and oats; and often-overlooked vitamins and minerals. I wanted to eat for energy and not scarf down fake meat substitutes. I wanted to avoid the vegan stereotype of pale, weak, and extremely thin.

I explained my idea to Alex, almost apologetic in my approach.

"Hey there, guy."

He looked at me. "Are you talking to me?"

I was obviously not great at this. "What are your thoughts on veganism?"

"None, really."

"Well, what do you think about it? As a way of eating?"

He set down the novel he was reading. "I think of Birkenstocks and hippies and frolicking through meadows and dreadlocks and hairy armpits."

"Don't forget peace signs," I added. "There are always peace signs." Really, I wasn't helping my cause.

"Why do you ask?"

"I was thinking about . . . you know . . . becoming one."

"A hippie?"

"No, a vegan. A vegan who's definitely not a hippie."

"Why though?"

I laid out my reasons: I felt heavier than I ever had. I definitely didn't feel as healthy as when I was a vegetarian. Eating as much meat as we did was ridiculously expensive. I wanted to feel healthy and clear-headed. Not to mention the horrendous treatment to animals. Unless I could raise the animal myself, I didn't trust where it was coming from or how it was treated.

"I don't know," he said. "Wouldn't it be hard?"

"No. Not if we know exactly how to supplement. We could try it for a short time. See how we feel and reassess. Almost like a cleanse."

"Okay."

I pounced on him. "Really? You think you could give up meat?"

"Yes."

"And our Sunday night egg-white omelets?"

"Yes."

"And Greek yogurt, and turkey pasta? And Parmesan cheese? "

Instantly, I was regretting my decision. What would happen to our Friday Italian nights? Our Sunday night egg-white omelets from Tempo? Our chicken fajita nights? I realized so much of the food I ate had an emotion attached to it. But I loved the memories food created, not necessarily the foods I was eating.

"Maybe we should wait until after Thanksgiving. One last goodbye," I said.

"Do you want to do this or not?"

"Do you?" I shot back.

"I do if you do."

I chewed on my lower lip and shrugged. "I need a change."

"So let's try it then."

While Alex loves animals, his grandfather was a cattle rancher. Alex worked in numerous restaurants as a line cook, and butchering dead flesh did not bother him. This wasn't about saving animals for him, but feeling healthier. He also wanted to see if he could maintain his strength, size, and endurance as a rugby player with only plant-based proteins.

With our decision in place, we had one last Thanksgiving meal, and then began to wean ourselves off of meat and dairy, one item at a time. A period of detoxification occurred as our colons adjusted to our new diet. We lost weight effortlessly, while increasing our energy with plant-fueled foods. Surprisingly, we didn't miss the chicken, turkey, and salmon, or the expensive whey protein and egg whites. Instead of simply cutting these foods out, we had a plan in place. We replaced meat proteins with plant-based proteins like legumes and seeds and protein-rich grains. We weren't spending an extra 50 to 100 dollars every week on meat and eggs. We were eating more, but more of the right foods for our bodies.

Weight sloughed off. Muscle mass increased. Soreness dissipated. Strength soared. Alex lost 50 pounds and played an entire rugby season in the fittest shape of his life. After games, when he used to fall on the couch in a coma, he wasn't even tired. He was only fueled by Medjool dates pre-game and a healthy vegan shake post-game, and his teammates marveled at his newfound frame and abilities.

I saw dramatic shifts in my own health too. I lost weight and that sluggishness that I couldn't previously shake. I had no more aches and pains. I felt better and looked better with such minimal effort. I could accomplish excruciating physical feats with ease. It was an experiment with instant success. As with any new way of eating, however, we knew that instant success did not necessarily mean we should or could eat like this for a lifetime. Time reveals how your eating is affecting your body. Many Americans can live on unhealthy diets, only to be reminded of it later in the form of diabetes, cancer, and numerous other diseases down the line. So it's *imperative*—especially when choosing a plant-based diet—that you know what you're doing, how to tweak your diet, and how to get all the vital nutrients that will lead to a healthy, happy life. What works for you today might not work for you five years from now, so be flexible. Be attentive to how you feel at any given time.

Three-Pronged Approach to Power Vegan Eating

As with any new habits, it often helps to have some principles to follow. Alex and I live our lives by the following three principles, each and every day. Living by these principles doesn't mean you have to give up meat or dairy. It's not about cutting foods *out*, but what you can do to add healthier habits *in*. Read and implement as you see fit—this is your body and your life. These principles will change your life (and make every day so much easier).

1. PAY ATTENTION TO HOW YOU FEEL

One of the most important things I ask my clients to do is to pay attention to how they feel after they eat. After assessing a few days' worth of typical eating, we pinpoint culprits, such as too many processed foods, too many hours between meals, or too much alcohol, salt, or convenience food. I help clients figure out why they eat the way they do and, more importantly, how they feel after they eat their typical fare.

Before you change the way you eat, ask yourself the following questions. Track your eating for a day or two, noting how you feel, and then examine each of the questions below separately.

Are you energized? Monitor your energy level after you eat. Do you feel an immediate surge followed by a crash? Or do you feel tired right off the bat? Are you more even-keeled—not too energized, but not depleted either? Do you feel energized in the mornings as opposed to the afternoons? While other factors can affect energy levels, it's important to pay close attention to what foods you are eating when your energy surges as opposed to when it plummets. And while you might feel a huge burst of energy after a large cappuccino and a sugary muffin, chances are you will probably crash in a few hours. If you are a caffeine addict, try cutting back a bit to see if you actually have more energy, not less.

Are you tired? If you become exhausted after highly processed meals, then you need to evaluate how those foods are affecting you. The same goes for dairy, meat, sugar, and caffeine. Do you feel great for a little while and then crash? How do you feel after having a highly processed meal versus a meal with fresh, unprocessed plant ingredients? A big salad versus a giant pasta dinner? Once you get a handle on how you feel, you can make successful tweaks to your diet to boost energy.

Do you get a stomachache? Are you bloated? If you become bloated or get a stomachache, you are probably eating a food or foods that don't necessarily agree with you. Though the offending culprits are usually dairy or wheat, any number of foods could negatively affect your system. See the sections on bloating and allergies in Chapter 11 for more information.

How do you really feel? Always ask yourself when you go to eat: How do I feel? How will I feel? How do I feel right now? Is this what I really want to eat? Healthy changes don't mean switching to low-fat, fat-free, low-carb, or low-calorie fare. They also don't mean counting calories or taking away foods you love. They are simply about eating foods that make you feel good. If a piece of cake makes you feel fantastic, then go for it. But, if you really pay attention to how you feel directly after, 20 minutes after, and even two hours after, you will start to get the messages your body is sending you.

Your body sends all the signals you need on a constant basis. All you have to do is tune in.

2. EAT PLANTS

While I'm not here to enforce a vegan lifestyle, we have grown up in a world where we eat far too much meat and dairy. It's simply the way we've been raised: The cow is the star.

However, we don't live in a time like our grandparents or even our parents, when animals were given more organic feed than they are now; when they weren't factory-farmed; when milk went through a few hands straight to a glass bottle and then to a doorstep, instead of through hundreds of factories and processes to cheap plastic jugs, all to be stored on some random shelf in the supermarket.

While it's not about the morals or ethics of eating meat for everyone—there will always be those who roll their eyes at vegetarians, and there will always be those who are passionate in their quest to not eat meat—we all need to think about the quality of our food. What has that animal eaten; how was it treated; was it packed tightly with other sick animals; what parasites did it have; how was it killed, "cleaned," and packaged? How long has it been sitting, dead, in the back of a truck, in a glass container, or in a package, touching other meats, before it was wrapped up by blood-soaked gloves to be thrown into a shopping cart and taken home to sit in your refrigerator or freezer? And, once it's ingested, what happens when that flesh interacts with your cells?

Just think before you eat. Figure out where your food comes from and most importantly, how it makes you feel. But regardless of what you eat, we can all use a little more green in our lives.

I hear the phrase "I hate vegetables," over and over again, and I am always baffled by it. What veggies do you really hate? And why? Perhaps you don't like vegetables because your body is not used to them, or you weren't fed veggies as a child (or vegetables were crammed down your throat and now you have an aversion to them). But, you can change this at any time. We are incredibly adaptable creatures.

All of our tastes are learned. We can just as easily unlearn them (yes, really). Do you ever wonder why kids' menus are the way they are? Why children love macaroni and cheese and pizza and chicken tenders? It's not because kids are naturally picky eaters. It's simply become standard for kids to eat this way because it's the food they are introduced to.

Our habits start young, but we can break them anytime. We can expose ourselves to healthier foods whenever we want to. Try this: When you walk into the grocery store and see the colors of the rainbow lining the produce shelves, see if you can spot five fruits and five vegetables that you enjoy. Since fruits and veggies are full of cancer-fighting compounds, they literally turn your body into a fighting machine.

If you load up on fresh produce, you *will* notice a difference in the way you feel. So start small. Start with one vegetable or fruit per week, and each week, make it a goal to try something new. Prep a big salad for the week. Take those leftover veggies in your refrigerator and blend them to make a healthy soup. Or pop a handful of spinach or kale into a smoothie for an extra dose of vitamins and minerals. It's about finding easy ways to get more plants into your diet every single day.

3. FIGURE OUT WHAT FOODS YOU LOVE AND LEARN HOW TO MAKE THEM HEALTHIER

It's not realistic to tell someone who loves pizza, pasta, or ice cream to just cut these foods out of their diet forever. If you're addicted to cigarettes, you can cut out cigarettes. If you're addicted to alcohol, you can cut out alcohol. Why? Because you aren't *required* to have them for survival every day. Food is one of the hardest components of any lifestyle to get right because we *must* eat food to survive.

It can sometimes feel like you are losing an uphill battle. I often walk into the grocery store and think, "Why isn't there just one brand of oatmeal? One type of quinoa? One kind of almond butter?" It's overwhelming to look at the shelves lined with hundreds of the same item. Which do you choose? What are you supposed to eat? What do those labels *really* say? Should I trust advertisers? (The answer to that last question is always no.) From my experience, if it comes in a plastic bag, a can, or a box, it's probably not in your best interest to purchase. Of course, there are exceptions to this rule, but it's a general one: *If it comes from a plant, eat it. If it was made in a plant, don't.*

But what if everything you love comes in a package, or you just can't resist your cravings? Often we think a good solution is to just go to the store and buy a low-fat, sugar-free version. But before you purchase your beloved item, you need to take a look at the ingredients. Are there words you can't pronounce? Then you don't want them in your body. Period. Lower-fat and lower-sugar items are usually packed with chemicals (check out the labels), and more and more companies are stamping "trans fat free," "made with natural ingredients," or "gluten free" on their labels to make you *think* they're healthier. But use common sense. If a box of Trix claims it's made with whole grains, okay. But what *else* is it made with? Don't be a blind participant in your health.

So, what do you do when you get a craving, or you know you aren't willing to give something up? You are going to make a healthier version using the recipes in this book, and you are going to love them more than the original. Love cookies? Try a flourless recipe. Love pasta? Pasta is a refined grain, which uses semolina flour and consists of empty calories that can often leave you tired. So try quinoa pasta or brown rice pasta, which are full of fiber, protein, and more nutrient-rich ingredients. Love mac and cheese? Make your own "cheesy" sauce from cashews, coconut oil, nutritional yeast, and tahini (see recipe on page 207). Love ice cream? Try a delicious nondairy version that will blow your mind (page 230). *Power Vegan* is never about deprivation. It's about making smarter choices *and* satisfying your cravings at the same time.

Reality Check

According to 2011 reports, over 25.8 million adults *and* children in the United States have diabetes—that's over 8 percent of the population. Complications of diabetes include heart disease, stroke, high blood pressure, blindness, kidney disease, nervous system disease, and even amputation.[4] Some potential causes of type 2 diabetes and other illnesses that plague the US population? Overconsumption of meat, dairy, alcohol, and processed foods, as well as gross inactivity.

In an era of indulgence, it's time to bring a consciousness to our meals and our snacking. Why? Because we are a population that is murdering itself with food. Massive portions, rushed meals, drive-throughs . . . is this love for ourselves and our health? No. Love for food means loving your body, recognizing every small morsel that enters your mouth, and more importantly, recognizing *why* you are eating these specific foods. What are you eating for nourishment, and what are you eating for comfort? Does that bite have a purpose or is it just a habit? If it is a habit, it can be broken. You're the one who controls your health—no one else.

So, think about it: Why do you eat the fried chicken? The heavy cheese? The mounds of processed food? Because it tastes good? Compared to what? Why does it taste good to you? Is it texture, flavor, or both? At what point did you learn to reach for these unhealthy foods? Is this adding longevity? Is this enhancing your years?

To enjoy healthy food doesn't mean to go without what you love. It just means slightly altering your preferences. Really think about your habits. Examine them. See where you can make improvements.

It's time to take your life back, and that begins with learning to love food—but they must be the right foods for you. I can't tell you what the right foods are for your body, but I can give you the tools and recipes to try to help you get there.

The keys to success? Start thinking simpler. Start thinking fresh. Ask yourself: What is the simplest way to get healthy food *today*? What will my activity level be *today*? What am I stressed about today? Am I tired? How do I feel, and what do I *really* need?

So, take it back to basics. Your body, your medical bills, your health, and your family will thank you.

SELF-ASSESSMENT: FIGURING OUT YOUR FOOD

Take a few minutes to answer the questions below. Be as specific as possible. Really think about each question, and pay attention to your responses. They will provide all the tools to make small, effective changes going forward.

1. *Would I say my diet is good, or could it use improvement? Explain.*

2. *How many times per day do I eat? How many hours apart are my meals? Is this consistent, or do I eat at different times every day?*

3. *Do I often feel tired? Energetic? When do I notice my periods of fatigue or energy spurts?*

4. *How do I feel after I eat highly processed foods versus fresh foods?*

5. *How do I feel when I eat out versus when I cook at home?*

6. *Do I have any food allergies?*

7. *What are my favorite foods?*

8. *What foods do I not like or will I not eat?*

9. *Do I get cravings? Sweet? Salty? When do these cravings strike?*

10. *How many veggies do I get per day? Fruits? Beans? Grains? Seeds? Nuts?*

11. *How much meat do I eat every day?*

12. *How do I feel when I eat a meat-based meal versus a plant-based meal?*

13. *How much dairy do I get on a daily basis? How do I feel after I eat dairy?*

14. When do I go grocery shopping? How many times do I go per week?

15. Am I a meat eater? A vegetarian? Am I interested in learning more about a plant-based life? If so, what are my concerns about leading a plant-based life? (Be specific. Is it that I won't get enough protein, that I feel my options will be limited, that I won't be able to eat out or socialize? Explain.)

16. Do I have children? Am I interested in improving their eating as well?

17. If I have children, what foods do they like? When were they introduced to those foods?

18. How often do I drink alcohol?

19. How often do I cook? Do I enjoy cooking? Would I be willing to cook if it took 20 minutes or less?

20. How many days per week do I eat out? What are my favorite types of restaurants?

21. What's my favorite meal of the day?

22. Do I like salads? Vegetables? Which vegetables do I particularly like? In what form do I usually eat my veggies (salads, steamed, grilled, sautéed, soups, smoothies, juices, etc.)?

23. What food(s) can't I live without?

24. What, if any, are the biggest hindrances for me to keeping what I see as a healthy way of eating?

25. In terms of healthy eating, what am I not willing to do? (Examples: cook, go to the grocery store, give up alcohol, etc.)

|||||||||||||||||||||||||||||||||||||||||||||||||||||||||||||||||||||||||||||||||||||||||||||||||||||||||||||||||||||||||||||||||||||||||||||||||||||||||||||

EVALUATE YOUR ANSWERS

1. If your diet could use improvement, figure out the culprits. Do you consistently skip breakfast? Eat lunch out every day? Indulge in huge dinners? Have a sugary coffee drink at 3:00 p.m. every day? Identifying your pitfalls can help you swap these habits with healthier ones. (See Chapter 12 on common obstacles to a healthy life.)

2. Our bodies like routine. If you eat at different times every day, the body experiences undue stress. It can start to kick its fat storage mechanisms into gear if you go too long without eating. Some people do better on three meals per day and others do better on five, so figure out what makes you feel best. If you only eat two to three times per day and get extremely tired, you might need some high-energy snacks to keep you stoked for daily activities. If you eat well one day then have a stressful day the next and go six or seven hours without eating, you are setting your body up for major stress. Try to get on some sort of eating schedule. Pack snacks to bring to work. Drink water, and don't ever skip meals.

3. Be an observer of your energy. When do you feel your best, and when do you feel tired? Is it related to food, stress, lack of sleep, or all of the above? While our energy can shift daily, try to pinpoint how specific energy changes are related to your food intake. Chances are, you will find some patterns. Do you always get tired after eating bread? Do you feel energized after a green juice? Jot down the foods that make you feel great and the ones that don't on any given day. Experiment with different foods to see what works best.

4. If you eat chips, cookies, pasta, and convenience foods one day, and then more wholesome foods the next day, you should be able to tell a difference. While it's not realistic to eat "perfectly" all the time, try to make the bulk of your meals from the fresh, whole foods described in Chapter 2, and not from a box or can.

5. Restaurants load food with salt and oil. Even when you think you're eating well, you're probably not. Figure out the meals you adore at your favorite restaurants and try to replicate simpler, healthier versions at home. If you're not willing to cook, ask your server how each dish is prepared and have it made according to your specifications. Follow the other tips for restaurant dining on page 91, and whenever you can, try to limit eating out to a few times per week.

6. Though you may not have any known food allergies, certain ingredients could still affect you. While gluten-free diets are all the rage, most individuals who partake of this way of eating do not have celiac disease (a disorder that causes a severe autoimmune reaction to wheat and gluten). Instead, they simply feel better without gluten. Are you one of those people? Do you do better without soy, nuts, or dairy? You can omit a food for 10 days and then reintroduce it to see if you notice any specific difference. You might even discover an allergy you weren't aware of in the process.

7. Make a list of your favorite foods and see how you can make them healthier. Do you eat your favorite foods out of habit, or because you really enjoy the taste? What happens when you replace them with something similar, or take a break from them? Don't be afraid to try new things.

8. In terms of what you don't like, think about the healthy foods you won't touch. Do you hate veggies? Maybe try to dip them in some healthy hummus. Does that make a difference? Browse through the recipes in this book and see what appeals to you. See if your "off limits" foods can be altered somehow. If not, concentrate on a few fresh, whole foods that you do like or are willing to try.

9. Cravings are tricky and can usually be associated with stress, lack of sleep, or sheer habit. Note for a week when your cravings strike and what they are for. Then peruse Chapter 13 and the section on cravings in Chapter 12 to see if you can quell your cravings with a healthier version.

10. Sometimes we overestimate the healthy foods we eat. If you only get one or two servings of veggies per day, make veggies your first priority. Jot down how much of any one food you get per day, using a handful as a portion size, and, as you read on, see where your diet could use tweaking.

11. Note how much meat you eat every day. Do you feel good when you eat meat? Perhaps try to swap some meat with beans or other plant-based proteins to see if you notice any difference, especially in energy and digestion.

12. Compare eating a typical meat-based meal to eating a plant-based meal. Do you have more or less energy? Is your digestion better? See what feels best to you.

13. Many people don't think they eat a lot of dairy, but when they study what they eat, they're surprised to find a little milk here, some cheese there, some yogurt in the morning or afternoon, and a slew of dairy hidden in other products. There is a common misconception that you must eat dairy to get enough calcium, but in fact, dairy is quite hard to digest (see Chapter 4). You don't really know how you feel without dairy until you cut back. Chances are, your digestion will improve, your skin will improve, you might lose that stuffy nose or that phlegm in your throat, and you will probably drop a few pounds in the process.

14. Note the times and days you go grocery shopping. Are these times and days working for you? If so, keep doing what you're doing. If you could use some improvement, whether it's having a more efficient shopping list or a better budget, use the tips on page 93 to come up with better ways to get your shopping done.

15. If you're slightly interested in learning more about a plant-based life, examine your reservations. Write them down, and then use this book as a guide to slashing those concerns (or jump to the sections that address your specific concerns—for example, Chapter 3 discusses how to make sure you get enough protein when eating a plant-based diet). See if you can tackle your concerns one at a time to come up with a way of eating that works best for you.

16. First, look at what your children eat. Do they eat out of convenience, are they picky, or do they eat what you eat? Do they consistently order off the kids' menu, and if so, why? Childhood is a wonderful opportunity to dose up on healthy food to ensure a healthy life. Whole foods should be the bulk of any child's diet, instead of processed convenience foods (for more on how to feed children the proper foods for their growing bodies, see Chapter 7). Though they might seem picky, they may not have been introduced to many healthy foods. Start small, with a few fresh fruits and vegetables or even a morning smoothie, to see where their diets might improve. Kids need nutrients too. Seeds, grains, legumes, and produce—these are all incredibly important for building a healthy foundation for a long life.

17. Jot down all the foods your children like. Have they always liked those foods, or are their preferences the result of who they hang out with, the school they go to, their family meals? If they tend to love unhealthy foods, use the tips in this book to make healthy swaps the kids won't even notice. There are sneaky ways to improve nutrition, even with pizza (see recipe on page 217) or mac and cheese (see recipe on page 207). And if you don't think it's important, think again: Their moods, skin, and internal health can drastically change just by altering their meals.

18. Jot down how many drinks you have per week. What are you drinking? How do you feel after? Try to aim for a glass of water before any alcohol. Stick to clear liquor or a glass or two of red wine, and try to limit to just a few days per week whenever possible.

19. Cooking isn't for everyone, but it can be easy, fun, and less expensive than eating out. Think about what you prepare and when, or if you don't cook, why you have an aversion to it. If you're curious, aim for some of the easy, quick recipes in Chapter 13 to see how delicious and fuss-free cooking can be.

20. Note how often you eat out and what you gravitate toward. Chinese? Mexican? Italian? Fancy restaurants? Tapas? There are ways to ensure what you're ordering is healthy if you ask the right questions. Or you can try to replicate some of your favorite dishes at home to save money and your waistline. See more tips for eating out in Chapter 5.

21. Pinpoint your favorite meal of the day and really make that matter. Have 10 recipes you can recycle, add to, or shift slightly, so you are really savoring every bite. If you love breakfast or lunch, feel free to indulge a bit more and taper off at night, since we are usually more sedentary in the evenings. If dinner is your favorite, try to fill your plate with colorful produce. Eat slowly and try to make healthier choices. If you insist on heavy dinners, go for a walk afterwards.

22. Concentrate on what you like and, from there, look at how you are getting your veggies. If you eat the same salad every day, perhaps it's time to shake things up. Aim for variety. If you like kale, try collards or mustard greens. If you like zucchini, opt for butternut squash or yellow squash. If you like salads, dress them up in a different way. Branch out and see what you can introduce into your diet.

23. Make a list of your top five "can't live without" foods. Figure out how often you eat them, and when. Then use the recipes in this book or look up some other options to introduce slightly healthier versions of your favorite foods.

24. We all screw up. Think about when, how, and why you fall off the wagon, or what holds you back from eating the way you really need to. Then come up with tangible solutions to help you avoid these hindrances or roadblocks. Use the tips and tools in Chapter 5 to combat any excuse.

25. Knowing what you're not willing to do will go a long way to help you succeed. List what you are absolutely unwilling to give up or do, and then figure out ways around those issues.

Look at your answers. Study them. See where your issues are, and, as you read this book, pay attention to where you might be able to improve. Use these answers as a guide as you read on, figuring out tangible ways to solve even the toughest eating issue.

Bottom Line

Knowing your issues with food intake is half the battle. Being extremely honest about the reality of your wants, needs, and habits can set you up for the kind of healthy lifestyle you want to achieve. But knowing what *you* need is the most important thing—not what anyone wants or needs for you.

QUICKEST WAY TO ENSURE SUCCESS: WRITE DOWN WHAT YOU'RE *NOT* WILLING TO DO IN TERMS OF A HEALTHY LIFESTYLE.

CHAPTER 2

Best Power Foods

"Never order food in excess of your body weight." —ERMA BOMBECK

Our bodies are extraordinary. We have the capacity to create, heal, live, and die, while experiencing a host of ups and downs in between. Historically, we knew what to eat and the proper amounts, much like animals. We were satisfied by unprocessed, natural foods. There were no gyms. There were no complicated jobs. Our lives were truly active. Hundreds of years ago, we didn't even know what crackers or cookies or potato chips were. The concept of fast food was inconceivable. We ate what was in season. Our bodies were generally much more in tune with what we needed and when.

Joshua Rosenthal, in his book *Integrative Nutrition*, tells a story of going to India during the winter and loading up on fruits at a market. He'd bought too many, and when he brought them back to where he was staying, he offered a guard a piece of fruit. The man said no. "I don't eat fruit in the wintertime, because the weather gets cold at night."

This man knew that fruit was a cooling food, and he didn't have to read a diet book to find that out. Fruits reduce your body temperature. According to Eastern medicine, eating lots of cooling foods in the colder months can lead to sickness. Rosenthal writes, "Our ancestors ate seasonally because they had no choice. Fresh greens grew in spring, fruit ripened in summer, root vegetables kept them going in the fall, and people relied on animal food to get them through the winter."[5]

Animals are smart. They know what to eat and when to eat it. We used to be smart, before highway transportation, factory farms, trans fats, and refrigerated trucks came into play. Now, we can eat anything at any time, whenever we want.

But by reaching for naturally powerful foods that will aid your body and not work against it, you can assure maximum health benefits with minimal effort.

I am going to provide a list of the top seasonal foods for your health, adapted from Rosenthal.[6] In addition to reaping the health benefits of eating seasonal foods, you will also save money by purchasing what's in season. But first, there are several other ideas to consider. I am a believer that all foods that come from the ground are beneficial for you in some way and that you don't have to follow any rule too closely when it comes to eating, but when in doubt, there are two principles you can follow to ensure that you are eating more like that of your ancestors. First, aim for unprocessed, organic food; and second, for food that is locally grown.

Though there's been much debate about nutritional value in organic versus conventional produce, one thing is clear: When you eat conventional produce, you are ingesting any pesticides that were used on that crop. When soil becomes compromised, the nutritional value of our produce can decrease. Using pesticides or antibiotics also drastically alters what we are ingesting (remember, you are eating those chemicals too). Soil conditions are often better with organic produce, and the food tastes better and is more flavorful.

What about local produce? When produce is shipped thousands of miles and then sits on a shelf, it loses many of its nutrients. The best produce is plucked directly from your garden—these foods are full of enzymes and nutrients ready to be devoured. But for those of us who can't have our own gardens, browsing local farmers' markets or being part of a food co-op is key. Always pay attention to where your food comes from to get the most nutritional bang for your buck. Just because it says organic doesn't mean it's fresh, so local might sometimes be the better option if you have to choose.

After the list of seasonal foods below, I've provided a list of my favorite power foods, which are packed full of antioxidants. Antioxidants are compounds that can help combat free radical damage and oxidation and can help protect our cells in numerous ways. Plant foods are abundant in antioxidants. (You may sometimes hear many of these power foods referred to as "superfoods." This term simply refers to any food that has an especially beneficial nutrient profile or set of health benefits.)

The foods listed are packed full of vitamins and minerals, but are not the only foods you should focus on. If it is a whole food (a food that comes from the ground or is in its unprocessed, natural state), go for it. Our bodies are made for variety, so change it up as often as you can. Reach for the colors of the rainbow. If you don't like something on this list, replace it. Always be willing to try something new.

FALL FOODS

Apples

Beets

Belgian endive

Brussels sprouts

Cranberries

Figs

Grapes

Mushrooms

Parsnips

Pears

Pomegranates

Pumpkin

Quince

Sweet potatoes

Swiss chard

Winter squash (acorn, butternut, buttercup, delicate, Hubbard, kabocha)*

WINTER FOODS

Chestnuts

Grapefruit

Kale

Leeks

Lemons

Oranges

Radicchio

Radishes

Rutabaga

Turnips

SPRING FOODS

Apricots

Artichokes

Asparagus

Avocados

Carrots

Cherries

Chicory

Chives

Collard greens

Dandelion greens

Fennel

Mangoes

Mustard greens

New potatoes

Peas

Rhubarb

Spinach

Spring lettuces

Strawberries

Sugar snap and snow peas

Watercress

SUMMER FOODS

Bell peppers

Blackberries

Broccoli

Cucumbers

Eggplant

Green beans

Nectarines

Okra

Peaches

Pineapple

Plums

Raspberries

Summer squash

Tomatoes

Watermelon

Zucchini

*Note: Despite its name, winter squash is technically best in fall, though it is still available during the winter months as well.

Top Power Foods

FRUITS

Berries: Packed full of antioxidants, these little cancer fighters combat oxidation and inflammation (both of which have been connected to cancer growth) and should be eaten daily. Choose from an array of berries in season.

Dates: One of my favorite pre-workout snacks, dates are immediately assimilated as energy in the body and provide the perfect amount of simple sugar for activity. Also used as a base for energy bars and nondairy ice cream, they take on flavors well and are packed full of vitamins, fiber, and minerals.

Grapefruit: Naturally full of vitamin C, this delicious fruit is also an inflammation fighter, a natural fat burner, and full of lycopene, a known "anti-tumor" phytonutrient.

Lemons: Lemon juice boosts immunity; helps throat infections, indigestion, and constipation; and is full of vitamins and protein. Packed with antioxidants, lemons can also help cleanse the organs and aid in relief from toothaches.

Limes: Used for ages for medicinal purposes, limes can help with digestion, eye care, ulcers, respiratory problems, and skin care. They are chock-full of antioxidants and vitamin C.

VEGETABLES

Beets: A natural detoxifier of the liver, beets thin the bile and improve small intestine function. Perfect in juices or in salads, beets also make a bright lip or cheek stain for those looking for natural makeup options.

Broccoli: A cruciferous veggie (part of the cabbage family), broccoli is high in fiber, low in calories, and nearly 40 percent protein. In soups, salads, or raw with a veggie dip, broccoli will keep you fueled and provide a whopping 135 percent of your daily requirement for vitamin C in just three ounces (85 g).

Collard greens: These natural cancer fighters rank among the highest on the power greens list. Steamed or raw, these hearty greens can be used as wraps instead of tortillas, and contain an extraordinary amount of vitamins K, A, and C, as well as folate, manganese, calcium, and fiber. Collards have even been found to brilliantly bind bile acids in the digestive tract, which helps lower the body's cholesterol.

Kale: This power green is rich in chlorophyll and alkalizes the body as well as oxygenating the blood, which leads to a reduction in fatigue. One cup (65 g) of kale provides 10 percent of your daily need for anti-inflammatory Omega-3s (see page 83), and this chewy, leafy green has been linked to natural processes of detoxification. Very versatile, kale can be eaten raw, sautéed, blended, juiced, or shredded and baked as tasty kale chips.

Sweet potatoes: Filling and nutritious, sweet potatoes are high in vitamins A and C as well as potassium and fiber. They can be steamed, baked, or made into chips or fries—and often taste much better than their white counterparts.

Zucchini: Though widely known as a vegetable in the culinary world, this versatile green is technically a fruit. Packed with fiber, zucchini is 95 percent water, which makes it extremely hydrating. A good source of vitamin B6, it is also easy on the digestive system. It's a perfect alternative to pasta and takes on the flavors of the food it's cooked with, filling you up with no caloric damage.

OTHER POWER FOODS

Apple cider vinegar: Apple cider vinegar is a star in the health realm—not only can it clean your house, relieve sunburns, cure yeast infections, improve digestion, and erase sore throats, it can help slash serious health risks. A natural anti-bacterial, apple cider vinegar helps lessen joint pain and heartburn, clear up skin problems, and promote circulatory health. It has everything from potassium and pectin to malic acid, calcium, and acetic acid. It also helps break down fats and helps your body use them instead of storing them.

Coconut oil: In addition to being a healthy fat that is used for energy rather than stored in the body, coconut oil has many other uses. Its anti-inflammatory, anti-microbial, anti-fungal, anti-viral, and antioxidant properties make it a true power food. Perfect for diaper rash or as an overall moisturizer, conditioner, or makeup remover, its uses extend beyond the kitchen.

Legumes: Legumes are one of the most perfect foods around. With one cup (about 177 g), you receive 16 to 28 grams of protein, as well as a ton of fiber and iron. You can choose from a variety of legumes, such as lentils, mung beans, pinto beans, black beans, kidney beans, peas, peanuts, or chickpeas, all of which are high in B vitamins.

Maca: An Incan superfood, this root (offered in capsules or powder form) comes from the plant family Cruciferae. It is instrumental in boosting immunity and increasing energy (and even libido). It contains vital B vitamins and vitamin C, can help ease premenstrual symptoms and chronic fatigue, and boosts endurance, increases fertility, and even improves memory.

Nutritional yeast: Yellow with a nutty cheese flavor, this inactive yeast (which is the only reliable non-animal food source for vitamin B12) gives you a full spectrum of essential amino acids and a balanced source of B vitamins (not to mention seven grams of protein per two tablespoons). Surprisingly similar to cheese, it can be used in place of Parmesan, sprinkled on popcorn or bread, or thrown on pasta sauce or salad. A little goes a long way, with just two tablespoons per serving.

Pea–brown rice–hemp protein powder: This power protein trio delivers everything a plant eater (or non-plant eater) needs and more. High in amino acids, protein, fiber, vitamins, and minerals, this powder trio will meet all of your dietary needs to replace a traditional protein shake. Hemp is the most readily available of the protein powders, and is considered a complete plant protein. It contains all of your essential amino acids and sports a plethora of antioxidants and Omega-3s and -6s, as well as magnesium, iron, and (of course) protein.

Pseudograins: Naturally gluten-free, these seeds offer a perfect balance of protein and vitamins. Buckwheat, amaranth, quinoa, wild rice, millet, and teff supply a variety of calcium, B vitamins, and fatty acids. Packed with protein, many pseudograins, such as quinoa, also have all eight essential amino acids. Per ½ cup (93 g) serving, there are 6 grams of fiber and a whopping 12 grams of protein. Most pseudograins can be boiled in water and ready in 20 minutes or less.

Raw, unsalted nuts (almonds, macadamias, pistachios, walnuts, etc.): Full of healthy fats, vitamins, minerals, omegas, and protein, raw, organic, unsalted nuts can add a huge nutritional boost to anyone's diet. A handful a day can stave off hunger and improve overall health. You also have the option of soaking nuts to unleash their enzymes for more health benefits and easier digestion.

Sea vegetables: More commonly known as seaweed, these veggies are the most nutrient dense around. Containing 10 times the calcium in cow's milk, they are a complete protein source (see page 66). A natural source of electrolytes, they are an endurance enhancer as well. Kelp, dulse, arame, kombu, and agar–agar are just a few. Check your grocery store for what's available.

Seeds (chia, flax, hemp, pumpkin, sesame, sacha inchi, etc.): Full of iron, healthy fats, amino acids, and protein, these little powerhouses are versatile, easily accessible, and a vital component in any diet. They are also natural inflammation fighters.

Sacha inchi seeds (which you may not have heard of), also sold under the brand name SaviSeed, contain 17 times more Omega-3s than salmon and 9 grams of complete protein.

Making the Most of Your Power Foods

Nuts and seeds are comprised of abundant vitamins, minerals, proteins, and natural oils that are beneficial to our bodies in countless ways. However, they are often difficult to digest. Soaking, germinating, dehydrating, or sprouting nuts, seeds, grains, and legumes unlocks the nutrients in these foods so that our bodies can more readily absorb them. The following is a handy soaking/sprouting guide to reach maximum nutrition and the best digestion possible.

Most of us won't have the time to take these extra steps, but do try them if you're curious and want to experiment. Too much work for you? Seek out sprouted grains, nuts, seeds, and legumes at health food stores. While they are a bit pricier, it can save you time. However, once you get into the practice of soaking and sprouting, you'll find it becomes just a natural part of your routine.

WHY SOAK?

Nuts, seeds, grains, and legumes contain enzyme inhibitors that can be rough on our digestive systems (especially when we eat too much at one time). In layman's terms, they are dormant. We need water to "wake them up" and release all those yummy nutrients. When these foods are soaked overnight, often in pure, salty water, the enzyme inhibitors are neutralized by the production of beneficial enzymes, which increase vitamin content in these foods and allow your body to easily digest and absorb them.

Some people suggest just soaking in water. Others suggest using a tablespoon of high-quality sea salt. I have tried it both ways and find both beneficial. However, I prefer to use sea salt whenever possible. Experiment to see what works best for you.

HOW TO SOAK NUTS, SEEDS, GRAINS, AND LEGUMES

Pour nuts, seeds, grains, or legumes into a large bowl. Sprinkle sea salt over them. Pour purified room-temperature water over them until they are completely covered and let them soak for the time recommended in the chart on pages 58 and 59. Cover the bowl with a cheesecloth, stocking, or paper towel whenever possible to keep bugs out (if you live in an area where this is a problem).

Once soaking time is finished, pour into a colander and drain. Rinse thoroughly with purified water a few times. Your nuts, seeds, grains, or legumes are now ready to use in any recipe or be eaten by themselves.

If you want to completely dry them out, this is where you can use a dehydrator for 12 to 24 hours (at temperatures usually around 116°F [47°C]) to dry and crisp them. Dehydrated nuts and seeds are perfect in recipes that require baking, as they are more nutrient dense and flavorful.

No dehydrator? No problem. Pour nuts and seeds onto a parchment-lined cookie sheet and place in the oven (no warmer than 150°F [66°C]). If your oven won't go that low, you can crack the door. While this is not the most energy-efficient of techniques, it should do the job.

Remove when the nuts and seeds are dry and slightly crispy. You can store in airtight jars until ready to use.

WHY SPROUT?

Sprouting is probably something you haven't given a lot of thought to, though you've probably eaten raw sprouts on top of a salad at some point in your life. Seeds, grains, and legumes have numerous nutritional benefits, but many of these benefits are kept from us by phytic acid, a form of phosphorous stored in plant tissues. Before a seed is germinated, this phytic acid binds with many vitamins, such as iron, copper, magnesium, and zinc, which makes it hard to absorb. Once they are sprouted, the phytic acid is neutralized and the seed becomes a living plant. The end result? Better absorbability and digestibility. If you have often had gas from legumes, soaking and sprouting helps with this as well.

Sally Fallon, author of the health tome *Nourishing Traditions*, explains, "The process of germination not only produces vitamin C, but also changes the composition of grains and seeds in numerous beneficial ways. Sprouting increases vitamin B content, especially B2, B5, and B6. Carotene increases dramatically—sometimes even eightfold."

HOW TO SPROUT

Though times may vary for sprouting (refer to the following chart), the method is similar for most seeds, nuts, grains, and legumes.

One easy method is to purchase a mason jar (or several) and fill the bottom third with what you want to sprout. Cover with purified water. On top of the jar, place a sprouting screen screwed into the lid. If you don't have a sprouting screen, use a cheesecloth kept in place by a rubber band, pantyhose, or even a little mesh screen cut to the size of the lid and attached to the jar. Let the jar sit overnight. If you don't have mason jars, glass bowls do the trick, as well as paper towels instead of the cheesecloth.

The next morning, keeping the cheesecloth or screen on, drain the water. Then fill the jar with water through the cheesecloth or screen. Rinse, keeping the cover on, and swish around to keep the air circulating. Tip the jar to let it drain after rinsing. Place the jar on its side on a counter for the remaining sprouting time. Repeat the rinsing process two to three times per day for the entire sprouting time.

Alternatively, you can just let the grains, seeds, nuts, or legumes sit, untouched, until they sprout ¼-inch to ½-inch tails. Then you can rinse and store in the refrigerator until ready to use.

Always make sure you are using clean jars or bowls and that the sprouts never smell moldy or look slimy. While some can be eaten raw, lightly steaming or cooking is usually best. You can even dry the sprouts in a dehydrator or oven and then grind to make flour.

SOAKING AND SPROUTING TIMES

INGREDIENTS	SOAKING TIME	SPROUTING TIME
ADZUKI	12 HOURS	3–5 DAYS
ALFALFA	8 HOURS	2–5 DAYS
ALMONDS	8–12 HOURS	12 HOURS
BARLEY	6 HOURS	3–4 DAYS

BUCKWHEAT	6 HOURS	2 DAYS
CASHEWS	2–2½ HOURS	N/A
CHICKPEAS	12 HOURS	12 HOURS
KAMUT	7 HOURS	2–3 HOURS
LENTILS	8 HOURS	12 HOURS
MILLET	8 HOURS	2–3 DAYS
MUNG BEANS	1 DAY	2–5 DAYS
NUTS (ALL OTHERS)	6 HOURS	N/A
OAT GROATS	6 HOURS	2 DAYS
PECANS	4–6 HOURS	N/A
PUMPKIN SEEDS	8 HOURS	1 DAY
QUINOA	2 HOURS	1 DAY
RED CLOVER	8 HOURS	2–5 DAYS
RYE	8 HOURS	3 DAYS
SESAME SEEDS	8 HOURS	1–2 DAYS
SPELT	7 HOURS	2 DAYS
SUNFLOWER SEEDS	2 HOURS	2–3 DAYS
WALNUTS	4 HOURS	N/A
WHEAT BERRIES	7 HOURS	2–2½ HOURS
WILD RICE	9 HOURS	3–5 DAYS

Note: If you want to soak all your beans, generally soak for 8–12 hours. Smaller beans will take less time, while large beans will take longer. Make sure not to oversoak before cooking. Most beans take anywhere from 40 minutes to 1½ hours to cook, while lentils take 20–30 minutes.

Taking the Extra Power Vegan Step: Eating Raw

You've probably heard a bit about raw foods or the raw food movement. And most likely, you don't want to partake in it. It might seem weird or impossible or completely non-conducive to your lifestyle. If you've visited a raw restaurant, it might have even turned you off with weird concoctions and tastes you weren't used to (I've been to a few of them myself).

In fact, it doesn't have to be weird to be healthy—this is rule number one. There are many ways to incorporate raw foods into your lifestyle that are delicious, simple, and won't compromise taste. And there are numerous reasons for choosing to eat raw (or even finding a 50-50 balance between cooked foods and raw foods).

All plant-based foods are alive with enzymes and other nutrients that can heal our bodies just by being eaten. These enzymes are often referred to as the "life force" of food, and many raw foodists praise their healing powers. Cooking food often destroys its nutritional value and leaves us feeling sluggish. Consuming cooked food can even lead in the long term to pancreatic damage. Because the pancreas has to churn out enzymes and sodium bicarbonate to break down cooked food, constantly eating huge cooked meals depletes these enzymes and taxes the body.[7]

We want to make the process of digestion easy on the body. Therefore, eating live foods to give us live nutrition makes sense, right? When we cook food at high temperatures, we are essentially eating "dead" food. Our bodies have to work much harder to digest cooked food than raw food. As authors Michaela Lynn and Michael Chrisemer, N.C., explain in their book *Baby Greens,* "Organically grown, raw, living foods provide the highest profile of truly usable elements while naturally conserving the digestive and immune functions."[8] Raw foods also keep the body alkaline, which is a great way to counterbalance the largely acidic American diet (see page 79).

Many ailments we experience come from the typical American diet (as previously discussed). By choosing fresh foods in their natural state, you can literally bring energy into your body.

This doesn't mean you have to commit yourself to eating raw 100 percent of the time. Most restaurants don't offer raw foods exclusively, and we all want the pleasure of dining out. But you can start experimenting with simple recipes and ingredients at home (or look at the handy tools in Chapter 15 to find resources for eating raw) and see how your body responds.

Chances are, you eat more raw foods than you think, especially in summer. If you drink smoothies, eat fruits, or have salads, or if you have begun to experiment with soaking and sprouting nuts, you are already on your way. Do you notice how you feel after these meals as compared to cooked foods?

If you want to eat raw, there are a few things to invest in to make your life a tad easier: a good blender, a dehydrator, a juicer, a food processor or coffee grinder, and a spiral cutter (also known as a saladacco), so you can turn virtually any veggie into a "noodle."

Eating raw can be easier than your typical diet in many ways. It takes the guesswork out of cooking or having to invest in tons of utensils, and you never have to use the stove or microwave. All meals can usually be prepared in minimal time with a small amount of effort.

But you *will* be going against the norm. As Lynn and Chrisemer explain:

> There is significant motivation to turn a blind eye to the discoveries made in living nutrition. Although we are seekers of health and wellness as an over-consuming nation, we are very attached (if not addicted) to the way that we eat; and . . . change to our way of life is seldom met without some resistance. Having even more profound of an influence on the nutritional information we read are perhaps the financial investments at stake. From meat and dairy to pharmaceutical products, many corporate structures' security depends on our eating habits and dietary beliefs remaining loyal to them.[9]

The authors explain that when we rediscover living, non-toxic nutrition (as found in organic, raw foods) we can heal and regenerate our bodies in ways we never knew before. Toxins are everywhere—in our food, our household products, and our environment. Rarely do we think about food as being toxic, but over time, when we continually eat canned goods and conventional meat, dairy, and produce, toxins build up in our bodies and can be hard to expunge. We are so used to eating cooked foods, foods in cans, foods that are dead and must be cooked to be deemed "safe;" foods that have been stored and sealed and packaged. These don't taste odd to us—in fact, it's raw foods that might taste weird, because they have been spared all the additives, preservatives, chemicals, and sweeteners.

But the beautiful thing about being human is that we can re-create our tastes and habits. Going raw is just one way to do this to feed both mind and body.

Regardless of whether you venture into the land of raw foods, plant foods can be incorporated into any diet to boost your health (see Chapter 15 for more raw resources and appliances). Use your judgment and experiment to see what works best.

Bottom Line

In terms of power foods, do what feels best. While it's exciting to try new things, it might be more manageable to add just a few of these power foods at first to see how you feel and how they fit into your lifestyle. Next step? Maybe soak some seeds and nuts and then try sprouting. Then try to eat a few meals per week that are raw. Breaking a new, healthier lifestyle into manageable, daily steps is easier than tackling it all at once.

QUICKEST WAY TO ADD POWER TO ANY MEAL: EAT RAW.

CHAPTER 3

But Where Do You Get Your Protein?

"Do you think horses and elephants worry about not having any animal protein in their diet? Elephants are bigger and stronger than you."
—RUTH HEIDRICH, PHD AND VEGAN TRIATHLETE

Seventh grade. Cafeteria line.

The lunch lady stared at me, picking at what I assumed was a bald patch beneath her hairnet. "What'll it be, hon?"

"The burger," I whispered, as she slopped a thin, gristly patty onto my chipped blue tray. I finished my trek through the line, adding a brownie and a lukewarm box of milk. I sat at my usual table, replete with band geeks, all going over their written scales before practice.

I bit into the burger. Immediately, something hard yet fleshy rolled across my tongue. I spit the gristle into my napkin and pulled back the bun. Most of the bread had disintegrated onto the gray meat. A wad of mayo was the culprit—also lukewarm and currently melted into the doughy, meaty glue. Its scent invaded my nostrils. I swallowed the piece of offensive meat and pushed my tray away.

"That's it," I exclaimed. "I'm never eating beef again."

My friends looked at me and shrugged. "That's weird," Nick said.

"I think I'm going to throw up." I rose and ran to the girls' restroom, hugging the toilet that smelled like dirty maxi pads. I read the derogatory writing scribbled on the walls. The spelling was terrible, which made it even more insulting. I knew I wouldn't actually throw up my food (I'd seen enough television specials at that age about girls doing just that to know how unhealthy it was), but there, in that bathroom, I made a decision to stop eating beef.

That finality—that I could decide to eat something or not eat something—unlocked a self-discipline inside of me that comes in handy in many aspects of my life today. I made a promise, even there, at my nondescript middle school during a cafeteria lunch, that would later define my entire life and career.

Though I became a vegetarian at 13, I didn't completely know what I was doing or what I needed, and went back to eating meat (albeit temporarily) as an adult. Growing up, it was "normal" to think that if I wanted to be strong, I needed animal protein.

Where does this idea that we need so much animal protein come from? For hunters and gatherers, meat became a common staple when crops were dying. But in today's world, the amount of wasted meat, factory farming, and horrendous animal treatment is not only staggering and heartbreaking, it is unnecessary. We do not need animal protein to be healthy or maintain muscle mass. Yes, that's right—we don't *need* it. In fact, we are healthier without it. The truth about protein is this: You can get all of the protein you need from plant sources, and you can eat *more* of them than you could sources of animal protein. This way of eating is limit*less*, not limiting (and this is coming from a voracious former meat eater). But, as sensible as this approach seems, it's not the way things are done in our country. We have an obsession with centering our meals around animal protein, and if you don't include a slab of meat at dinner, it's often viewed as an incomplete meal.

The traditional American diet, which includes a serving of meat with nearly every meal, is not practiced in many countries in the world. In fact, many cultures (including regions of India and Asia) eat a largely plant-based diet and the health benefits of such a diet have been proven. Japan has the largest number of centenarians in the world. A report from the *Guardian* revealed that for the 50,000 centenarians alive today, plant-based diets have a large part to do with longevity and health.[10]

According to over 80 years of research by Dr. T. Colin Campbell as part of the China-Cornell-Oxford Project, one of the largest studies of nutrition ever conducted, cancer can literally be turned on and off just by altering protein intake. Campbell, a professor of biochemistry at Cornell University, found that the offending culprits were meat and dairy. He and his colleagues write,

Casein, which makes up 87% of cow's milk protein, promoted all stages of the cancer process. What type of protein did not promote cancer, even at high levels of intake? The safe proteins were from plants, including wheat and soy. Dietary protein proved to be so powerful in its effect that we could turn on and turn off cancer growth simply by changing the level consumed.[11]

In layman's terms, this means that by altering your protein intake to much lower than that of most Americans and altering the source of your protein, you can stop cancer growth. This is scientific research at work, not opinion (though it must be noted that this study was done on entire population groups and not individuals). The countries with the greatest statistics of longevity and health are those with the least amount of meat and dairy in their diets. Studies have also shown that excessive protein— especially animal protein—can cause elevated levels of ammonium in the reproductive tract.[12]

Not only are there health risks when we consume too much animal protein, but there are ethical implications as well. According to the *Livestock's Long Shadow* environmental and agricultural report, raising animals for food causes more global warming than all the cars and trucks in the world *combined*. Eating meat wastes resources as well. Ecologist David Pimentel notes in that same report that "[i]n terms of caloric content, the grain consumed by American livestock could feed 800 million people. Animal protein also demands tremendous expenditures of fossil-fuel energy—eight times as much for a comparable amount of plant protein."[13]

While this book isn't about the effects of the dairy and meat industries, it is about facts and habits. Ingesting animal protein is just one habit. Challenge yourself to think about why you eat the protein that you do. Is it because you were taught to do it? Or because you genuinely feel healthier with it?

Whatever your answer, we could all use more plant-protein sources. They are easier to digest than animal proteins, contain a host of vitamins and minerals often lacking in meat, and are *far* less expensive than their furry-friend counterparts.

Complete Proteins

The worry remains that if you don't eat meat, dairy, or eggs, protein deficiency is imminent. Amino acids, a vital component of muscle and brain health, have received much discussion in recent years. It's been argued by numerous dietitians, health gurus, and even doctors that you can't get enough of the right kind of protein as a vegetarian or vegan, because plant-based foods don't contain all the essential amino acids that meat and dairy do. But, in fact, most vegetables contain not only the essential amino acids, but *all* of the amino acids.[14]

To understand the way our bodies use and process protein, first you need to understand the essential aminos, so called because your body can't produce them and must get them from outside sources. They are:

Histidine	Phenylalanine
Isoleucine	Threonine
Leucine	Tryptophan
Lysine	Valine
Methionine	

Complete proteins are those that contain all of these essential amino acids. All proteins are made up of amino acids, whether you are eating a chicken breast or a mung bean; it's their amino acid profiles that are different.

Because non-animal protein sources can be low in a few amino acids (like lysine and methionine), they have gotten the reputation for being low in protein. While animal proteins contain the nine essential aminos (and are therefore considered complete proteins), plant proteins differ slightly. Plants have varying amino profiles. While some can be low in the essential aminos, others are abundant. So if you only eat cereal and soda, you aren't going to be getting what you need. Or if you only eat legumes or fruits, for instance. This stands true of any diet. But in fact, you can get everything you need from a plant-based diet. Eating a diet with a large variety of plant foods is the key to making up the deficit. When you combine grains, legumes, nuts, seeds, and veggies (as you would in most meals), these foods become complementary and provide all essential aminos.

This doesn't mean you have to pay attention to how you pair your foods (that would be exhausting). Instead, focus on getting a variety of plant-based proteins every day and you will be covered. There are several plant-based foods that do contain all essential aminos, however: soy, quinoa, hemp, chia, and chlorella, to name a few. This doesn't mean you have to gorge yourself on tempeh, tofu, soy milk, quinoa, and seeds every single day. Just one cup (248 g) of tofu or a few tablespoons of hemp or chia cover your essential amino bases, so you can see how easy it actually is to get what you need.

But what if you have an aversion to soy? Stick to a large variety of soy-free foods to cover all your bases, such as lentils, almonds, chickpeas, tahini, seeds, peanuts (remember that peanuts are a legume!), peas, and rice.

While it is harder than most people think to become protein deficient, you *can* become deficient if you don't know what to eat (and no, eating a bunch of fake meat alternatives is not the answer).

Worried about how much protein you need? Diets with 10 to 15 percent protein (versus 30 percent, as some Americans consume) are the healthiest.[15] A safe calculation is as follows:

your weight x .36 (add 10 grams if you are pregnant)

Your Plant-Based Protein Sources

The following foods will help you curb cravings, keep you full, and give you the same amount of protein, vitamins, and minerals per serving you would find in meat (if not more). Individualize your protein sources based on your own preferences and needs.

IF YOU EAT CHICKEN OR TURKEY, TRY: SEEDS

Seeds provide numerous vitamins and minerals, and yes, even protein. Whether it's pumpkin, sunflower, chia, flax, sacha inchi, or hemp seeds, you are getting around eight grams of protein per ¼ cup (33 g), along with countless nutrients. You're getting essential amino acids and Omega-3s (and you don't have to cook them). Simply toss on salads, in smoothies, or in soups for a powerful dose of vitamins and protein. And contrary to popular belief, "grains" such as quinoa (which is a complete protein) and wild rice are actually pseudograins, or seeds (see page 55). Quinoa totes 20 grams of complete protein per one dry cup (170 g). All you have to do is boil some water, toss the quinoa in, and simmer for 15 minutes.

IF YOU EAT BEEF, TRY: LEGUMES

What are legumes? They are the edible parts of plants in the legume family, such as peas or beans. Legumes can include beans, dry seeds, and even what we think of as vegetables (contrary to popular belief, *all* plants have protein). Per one-cup (177-g) serving of beans (kidney, black, garbanzo, or lentils), you are getting 16 to 28 grams of protein, along with iron, a good source of fiber, and negligible fat. They are also high in B vitamins, rich in antioxidants, and low on the glycemic index. (The glycemic index ranks foods based on how they affect blood sugar levels.)

Use in soups, chili, or salads, or shape into patties and have in place of a burger. Dried beans are best (soak overnight and then cook the next day). If you don't have time to soak and cook dry beans, always look at the can or box label. Opt for those with the least amount of sodium. Certain companies, such as Eden Foods, now offer BPA-free cans for toxin-free cooking. Fig Food Co. and other companies are now also offering organic boxed beans, so you can avoid cans altogether.

IF YOU EAT FISH AND EGGS, TRY: HEMP

Hemp is an amazing complete plant protein full of essential fatty acids, fiber, and vitamins B and E. It is also one of the few plant sources to contain all of your essential amino acids. Because it comes in many forms, you can experiment to see what you most enjoy.

You can purchase hemp in the form of a protein powder for shakes, seeds to sprinkle on oatmeal or salads, or even in the form of milk (which can also be made on your own by grinding hemp seeds and water and then straining through a nut bag). Per one serving (only 1.5 tablespoons), hemp contains five grams of protein. One cup of hemp protein powder has a whopping 20 grams of protein. Hemp is much more affordable than eggs or fish per serving, is easier to digest, and boasts a better nutritional profile. Still want the texture of scrambled eggs? You can scramble up some tofu and toss in some hemp seeds to get a double dose of complete protein.

Bottom Line

Experiment with different forms of protein to see what makes you feel best. Instead of planning your meal around a piece of meat, you can make veggies, grains, legumes, and seeds the star players.

You might surprise yourself by feeling a difference in energy, since your body has to work so much less to break these plant proteins down. You will be left with more fuel for daily activities instead of digestion. The best part: Plant proteins are significantly cheaper than meat, they last longer, and they are easier to incorporate throughout the day.

Other surprising places to get protein?

Avocados: 7 to 10 grams of protein each

Broccoli rabe: 17 grams of protein in one bunch

Cocoa powder: 17 grams of protein in one cup (86 g)

Cooked spinach: 13 grams of protein in one cup (180 g)

Nutritional yeast: 16 grams of protein in one cup (192 g)

Soybeans: 14 grams of protein in one cup (172 g)

Split green peas: 26 grams of protein in ½ cup (73 g)

Teff: 26 grams of protein in one cup (192 g)

Spacing out your protein between meals should be more than enough to cover your protein bases. Virtually every food contains protein, especially greens. If you eat a variety of foods, you should be covered.

Worried about losing lean muscle mass? Don't be. You can maintain all your lean muscle, gain muscle, and be fitter than you ever were—all with plant protein.

QUICKEST WAY TO ADD PROTEIN: THROW LEGUMES OR SEEDS ON ANY DISH!

CHAPTER 4

Eat Your Vitamins

"It is no measure of health to be well adjusted to a profoundly sick society."
—JIDDU KRISHNAMURTI

Many people associate vegan diets with vitamin deficiency, but in fact, vitamin deficiency is a problem in many traditional American diets. Why? Because our food isn't as nutritious as it used to be. As a result, we are suffering from micronutrient deficiencies. Micronutrients are essential elements needed for life in small doses—in other words, vitamins and minerals. Due to poor eating and soil conditions, it's not uncommon for American diets to be lacking in micronutrients.

Deficiencies in vitamins and minerals can lead to a host of health problems, including obesity. If someone is consuming a poor diet that lacks vitamins and minerals, the appetite remains stimulated due to the body's attempt to make the individual keep eating until basic nutritional needs are met. Our bodies *know* what they need. They will keep attempting to eat until we give them antioxidant-rich foods with fiber, vitamins, and minerals.

Foods high in sodium and sugar with a high calorie density but low nutrient content don't trigger appetite sensors to signal fullness. (So, the next time you are starving after eating an extra-large pizza, you'll know why.)

There are several vitamins and minerals that are not abundant in plant-based foods and need to be paid special attention, especially when entering the world of plant eating. Vitamins B12 and D, calcium, folate, iron, and zinc are the top contenders. Most people think they can down a multivitamin and be covered, but our bodies know the difference between a tablet and the real thing (though reaching for foods fortified with these micronutrients is still a step in the right direction). If you took a multivitamin or juiced 10 vegetables, which would be a better source of nutrients? Regardless of how easy it might seem to just opt for vitamins, aim to get your nutrients through whole foods and natural sources whenever possible.

The following are the most important vitamins to pay attention to when leading a plant-based life. While all vitamins and minerals are important, the following are often lacking in plant-based diets if not properly planned for.

Vitamin B12

Known as the energy vitamin, vitamin B12 is responsible for cell division, tissue synthesis, formation of red blood cells, and smooth muscle movement. It helps with the metabolism of fat and protein. It is also essential for a healthy nervous system and energy, especially if you exercise often. If you haven't paid much attention to this vitamin, it's a good idea to start.

Deficiency can lead to nerve damage or even heart disease (and can often go undetected for many years). Unfortunately, this vitamin, which is made by bacteria, is not abundant in plant food. It's easy to become deficient in vitamin B12 if you don't know where to look.

While there are numerous supplements on the market, our bodies don't often absorb these mega doses and will instead take in a small amount and excrete the rest. Many sources also debate which type of B12 is best: cyanocobalamin (used in supplements and fortified foods) or methylcobalamin (a form that doesn't need converting). Choosing a supplement that can be dissolved under the tongue or chewed is usually best.

You should aim to get 2.4 mcg per day. However, if you are taking a supplement, you might need a much higher dose than this (anywhere from 24–1,000 mcg, depending on how often you are supplementing) to ensure your body is absorbing the proper amount. If you don't know what ranges are right for you, you can get your vitamin B12 levels checked. However, if you eat a plant-based diet and don't eat the foods listed below, aim for a higher dosage to up your stores. A lack of energy can be another indicator that you might need a higher dosage. If you eat the foods on this list, feel energetic, and even take a vitamin, you should be covered.

BEST FOOD SOURCES OF VITAMIN B12

Chlorella*

Fortified nondairy milk

Fortified ready-to-eat cereals

Kombucha*

Nutritional yeast*

Sea vegetables*

Veggie "meats"* (These should not be your sole source for this vitamin, as they are still processed and often full of sodium.)

Fortified energy bars

Note: The foods on this list, with the exception of the fortified foods, contain negligible amounts of vitamin B12 and should not be considered substitutes for vitamin B12-rich foods. Because plant foods in general only contain trace amounts of this vitamin, vegans should always supplement accordingly.

Calcium

Calcium is used by the body in numerous ways. It is vital for building healthy bones and teeth. It aids in muscle contraction, cell membrane functions, clotting blood, and regulating enzymes. Ninety-five percent of the body's calcium is stored in the skeleton.

We are brought up thinking we must have dairy to get enough calcium (though we are the only species to drink another species' milk). But despite what the billion-dollar dairy industry would like you to believe, you don't have to ingest dairy to be healthy. In fact, our ancestors used to get large doses of calcium from leafy greens, not animals. Dairy is not only hard to digest, it makes our bodies incredibly acidic (see page 79) and actually leaches calcium from our bones. The United States, ironically, has the highest levels of osteoporosis in the world, despite having the highest dairy and protein consumption.[16]

Those who are lactose intolerant are left searching for calcium in other forms. From anywhere between 18 months and 4 years old, we lose 95 percent of the enzyme lactase, which is needed to digest lactose.[17] According to extensive studies by Dr. Samuel Epstein, MD, professor emeritus at the University of Illinois School of Public Health, our milk also contains bovine growth hormone (a genetically engineered hormone often given to cows), pus from infected udders, radioactive particles, PCBs (polychlorinated biphenyls, industrial chemicals that can cause a variety of health problems), and brominated flame retardants.[18] Many cows even have Johne's disease, a bacterial disease of the small intestine that has been shown in some studies to be connected to Crohn's disease in humans. So, there are infinite reasons to give it up.

However, calcium is finicky: to be properly absorbed, it has to be consumed in a two-to-one ratio with magnesium, which is not always the ratio in dairy products. To ensure you are getting the right ratio, focus on foods that are high in magnesium, such as squash, cocoa, flax, tahini, sunflower seeds, almonds, molasses, and edamame. The great news? Most of these foods are also high in calcium, ensuring the perfect ratios.

Calcium is easy to get if you're a plant eater, as many foods are fortified with it (orange juice, cereals, tofu, tempeh, soy milk, etc.) However, you can get all the calcium you need from non-fortified foods like plants and healthy grains. The recommended range varies from 800 mg per day for children to 1,200 mg per day for seniors. The average adult needs around 1,000 mg per day.

BEST FOOD SOURCES OF CALCIUM

Almonds	Dried fruit	Quinoa
Amaranth	Figs	Rhubarb
Apricots	Fortified nondairy milk	Sea vegetables
Bean sprouts		Soybeans
Blackstrap molasses	Fortified nondairy yogurt	Spinach
Bok choy	Fortified orange juice	Tahini
Broccoli		Tempeh
Brown rice	Fortified ready-to-eat cereals	Tofu
Brussels sprouts	Kale	Turnip greens
Cabbage	Mustard greens	Unhulled sesame seeds
Chia seeds	Navy beans	White beans
Collard greens	Okra	

While eating a broad spectrum of calcium-rich foods is key, there are several factors that can hinder absorption, such as ingesting alcohol and caffeine; smoking cigarettes; and eating animal protein, salt, soda, many junk foods, and too much oxalic acid. Regarding this last one, while many leafy greens contain calcium, certain greens with oxalic acid (an acid found in plants that is potentially harmful for those with oxalate sensitivity) can hinder absorption (annoying, yes). Greens containing oxalic acid include spinach, Swiss chard, rhubarb, and beet greens. To avoid this problem, simply aim for a wide variety of greens, rather than too much of any one, to cover your calcium needs. It is also suggested that if you take a calcium supplement, you take it between meals for better absorption.

Vitamin D

This vitamin helps bones and teeth and is vital for skeletal development. It also helps the body absorb calcium. Known as the sunshine vitamin, vitamin D can be hard to get from plant foods and is best derived from direct exposure to UV rays. If you can, opt for 15 or 20 minutes of uninterrupted, unprotected sunshine daily on your arms, face, and legs. If you are going to be out in the sun longer, apply natural sunscreen. (Many practitioners of holistic medicine believe that the chemicals in regular sunscreen actually promote skin cancer. Do your research and peruse all ingredients for anything you put on your skin. If you can't eat it, don't wear it.)

The recommended dosage of vitamin D is 10 mcg, or 400 IU, but if you feel you are lacking, aim for around 25 mcg, or 1000 IU, per day. It's important to note that there are two types of vitamin D: vitamin D3, which is derived from lanolin in sheep's wool or from fish oil; and vitamin D2, which is derived from yeast exposed to the sun. Most foods are fortified with vitamin D3, so search online or at your health foods store for plant-based vitamin D2 or D3.

BEST FOOD SOURCES OF VITAMIN D

Fortified nondairy milk (read all labels to see which brands have the highest amounts)

Nutritional yeast

Raw white mushrooms (exposed to UV rays)

Sun-dried shiitake mushrooms

Folate

Folate is a B vitamin found naturally in foods. In supplement form, it is referred to as folic acid. If you plan on getting pregnant, you can up your intake of folate even before you become pregnant to around 400 mcg per day, and to around 600 mcg once you are pregnant. Folate works in conjunction with vitamin B12 to help produce red blood cells. Most vegans and vegetarians get enough folate, but high intake of folate can often mask insufficient vitamin B12 on a blood test, so it's important to cover all your bases.

BEST FOOD SOURCES OF FOLATE

Dark, leafy greens

Legumes

Nutritional yeast

Orange juice

Pseudograins

Whole grains

Iron

Iron is all-important for facilitating red blood cell health. Enough iron ensures that the body is able to deliver oxygen-rich blood to the extremities. There are two types of iron: heme and nonheme iron. Plant foods contain only nonheme iron, which can be harder to absorb. Many individuals (primarily women) can become anemic when not ingesting enough iron-rich foods, or when menstruating. Therefore, it is important to ensure that you aim for high iron intake (either from heme sources, such as animal protein, or from a gentle vegan supplement, like those from New Chapter Supplements).

Generally, the recommended dosage is 18 mg of iron per day, but can be higher if you are pre-menopausal (as much as 33 mg). However, it's important not to get extremely high doses of iron, as too much in the blood can be toxic. If you can, skip the supplements (as they can be harsh on your system and back you up) and eat iron-rich foods instead.

Since iron is best absorbed with vitamin C, it's good to pair your iron-rich foods with foods high in vitamin C, such as strawberries, broccoli, collard greens, kale, Swiss chard, bell peppers, and citrus fruits. Eating iron-rich foods with calcium can actually decrease iron's absorbability, however.

BEST FOOD SOURCES OF IRON

Beet greens

Blackstrap molasses

Bran flakes

Dark chocolate

Dried beans and lentils

Dried fruit

Dulse

Kale

Kombu (this sea vegetable contains 38.6 mg per ½ cup [40 g] cooked—one of the best plant sources for iron)

Pumpkin seeds

Raw, whole cacao beans (1 ounce supplies 314 percent of daily iron needs)

Soybeans

Spinach

Split peas

Zinc

Necessary for growth and development, zinc allows the body to use dietary protein as building blocks for muscle regeneration. It also helps in proper immune function and countless enzymatic reactions. The standard suggestion for intake is around 11 mg per day, but some feel vegans should boost this to between 12 and 16 mg. Opt for a wide variety of foods that are good sources of zinc.

BEST FOOD SOURCES OF ZINC

Amaranth

Beans

Bran flakes

Brown rice

Buckwheat

Nutritional yeast

Nuts

Peas

Pumpkin seeds

Quinoa

Spinach

Tempeh

Tofu

Wheat germ

Wild rice

For all vitamins and minerals, rather than focusing entirely on supplements, try to aim for a variety of fruits, nuts, vegetables, grains, and seeds per day. This is the best way to ensure you're getting the proper nutrients. However, it's important to note that vitamin B12 and vitamin D need a bit of special attention. A small amount of sunshine and a quality B12 supplement are key.

What About the Rest?

If you eat a varied diet and pay attention to how you feel, chances are you'll get everything you need. Don't be afraid to try new foods on these lists to ensure you're getting all the nutrients your body requires.

In addition to "eating our vitamins" via whole foods, we also need to pay attention to whether our foods are alkaline or acidic, and how this affects us. American diets are largely acidic. When you eat a diet comprised mostly of acidic foods (such as meat and dairy), your body has to work hard to restore its pH balance, and will often leach minerals from bones in order to do so. Eating more alkaline foods donates minerals to the body. You should work to maintain a balance. We need a balanced pH level of 7.4 to even survive. So, think: acidic=leach; alkaline=donate.

If you want to know how your body responds to the foods you eat, you can pick up a pack of pH strips at any drugstore and test whether your body is acidic or alkaline. You can purchase strips to test your urine or saliva. Acidic conditions decrease the body's ability to absorb important nutrients. They prevent proper cell repair, and contribute to numerous health problems and disease. Even if you eat a diet rich in alkaline foods, but your body processes these foods as acidic—meaning it burns or digests them as acids—you might be out of balance.

If you want to err on the side of caution and incorporate more alkaline foods into your diet, aim to eat from the list of alkaline foods that follows.

ALKALINE FOODS

Almonds
Apple cider vinegar
Apples
Apricots
Avocado
Bananas
Beets
Berries
Carrots
Celery
Coconut (fresh)
Dark, leafy greens
Dates
Dried figs
Garlic
Grapes
Green beans
Kiwi
Lemons
Lettuce
Lima beans
Limes
Millet
Oranges
Papaya
Parsley
Pears
Pineapple
Raisins
Spinach
Spirulina
Sprouts
Strawberries
Tempeh
Tofu
Tomatoes
Wheatgrass
Zucchini

ACIDIC FOODS

Almond milk
Amaranth
Bacon
Barley
Beef
Beer
Black beans
Blueberries
Bread
Butter
Canola oil
Carob
Cashews
Cheese
Chickpeas
Cocoa
Coffee
Corn
Fish
Flax oil
Flour (wheat and white)
Hard liquor
Hemp seed oil
Ice cream
Kamut
Ketchup
Kidney beans
Lentils
Milk
Mustard
Noodles
Oats
Olive oil
Peanut butter
Peanuts
Pecans
Pepper

Pinto beans
Pork
Quinoa
Rabbit
Red beans
Rice (all)
Sesame oil
Soybeans
Soy milk
Sugar
Sunflower oil
Tahini
Turkey
Vinegar
Walnuts
White beans
Wine
Winter squash

Obviously, there are numerous healthy foods on the acidic side of the chart (and this is just a sampling of acidic and alkaline foods—you may find some charts with differing advice or suggestions). The fact that a food is acidic does not mean to avoid it; instead, balance it by eating a wide variety of alkaline-forming foods. Notice how you feel after eating alkaline foods versus acidic foods. Do you notice a difference? Feel more energy? Have better digestion? Also pay attention to how your food is prepared, and remember to aim for a large variety of vitamins and minerals with the foods you eat to maintain the best results.

Bottom Line

Even if you're not vegan, take a look at the foods you're eating. Are they full of vitamins, or mostly empty calories? Making nutrient-rich foods the bulk of your diet can cut supplement costs and provide you with a purer form of nutrition than synthetic replacements. Load up on alkaline foods and scan these lists to bulk up your vitamin and mineral profile with every meal.

QUICKEST WAY TO ADD VITAMINS TO YOUR DIET: EAT PRODUCE!

CHAPTER 5

Eat for Life

"Tell me what you eat, and I will tell you what you are."
—JEAN ANTHELME BRILLAT-SAVARIN

"I just can't lose those last five pounds."

I looked at my friend, who appears fit and trim to the rest of the world. She doesn't have five pounds to lose, yet she is convinced she does. We have been having this same conversation for the last *decade*—and no matter what I recommend, she sticks to her guns and self-bashes any chance she can. She has ventured into doing the Ironman, countless marathons, triathlons, adventure races, weightlifting, and even boxing. No matter what she does, her weight and body stay the same. She has a good job, albeit a stressful one. She makes great money, has a steady boyfriend, and has no debt. But, she is not happy. She is a bit of a self-sabotager and always seems to drum up drama in her personal life, especially when it comes to relationships.

She avoids carbs as though they are the devil, despite the fact that she is an endurance athlete. She keeps her focus on the scale, on what's on her plate, on how many calories she eats. She focuses on what she doesn't want to happen in her job, her relationship, and especially in her body, rather than what she *does* have.

In other words, she is stressed, which affects her weight, her attitude, and especially the hormones that can wreak havoc on overall health and fitness.

Chances are you have someone like this in your life. You might even see them at the gym, pounding away diligently, but never making any gains. Perhaps you know a yo-yo dieter or someone who always gives in to the latest fitness craze. You see their excitement as the diet works before the inevitable plummet into deprivation, followed by a slow descent into old routines and patterns. Perhaps this person is you.

Regardless, all these people have something in common: They must eat to survive. But how do you eat for life when life consistently gets in the way? No matter how many times I tell my friend to relax, to let go, to focus on the positive, her old routines and habits rear their ugly heads. It's in our nature. It's the way we are . . . or is it?

Five Hidden Culprits of Poor Health

We are all creatures of habit, especially when it comes to what we eat and why. Whether you've literally tried everything to lose weight but the pounds won't budge, you're undernourished and exhausted, or you have a sluggish colon, start by looking at these five hidden culprits to discover if you could be missing some obvious health signs. You never know where the culprit may be lurking.

YOU HAVE A DEPRESSED METABOLISM

Contrary to popular belief, your metabolism doesn't have to slow as you age. Though it's true that we experience a 2 to 4 percent decline in our resting metabolic rate with each passing decade after the age of 25, and on average, we lose about 5 pounds of lean body mass per decade from 25 to 65, this can be prevented in many ways. A decreased metabolism is from decreased *activity*, which leads to a slower, depressed metabolism, especially later in life.

A slow metabolism is lifestyle related, not age related. There are many scientifically proven responses to exercise that your body goes through, but one thing stands out: You can keep a healthy metabolism with plenty of activity. Muscle is metabolically active. The more lean mass we have, the better, especially later in life. We were not made to sit all day. So, start moving and don't blame weight gain on a slow metabolism. With activity and smarter choices, you can shift that metabolism and keep your energy revved and your weight healthy late into life.

YOU ARE SUFFERING FROM MICRONUTRIENT DEFICIENCIES

As discussed in Chapter 4, many American diets are lacking in micronutrients. Deficiencies in vitamins and minerals can lead to a host of health problems, including obesity. Making sure you are eating a diet with a wide variety of nutrients is key to staying healthy. Try to fill your plate with the colors of the rainbow instead of grays and browns.

YOU ARE EATING TOO MANY INFLAMMATORY FOODS

If you are active but constantly sore or suffering from nagging injuries, chances are it could be related to your diet. For example, often my clients experience nagging cramping and soreness despite a pretty "clean" diet. Upon closer inspection of their diets, I find they're ingesting way too many inflammatory Omega-6s in the form of corn, vegetable oils, and sunflower seeds. Therefore, the ratio of Omega-6s to Omega-3s is way out of balance. Switching the ratio to more Omega-3s (a natural inflammation fighter) and lowering the 6s gets things under control.

Many people suffer from chronic injuries or allergies and don't think about how the foods they eat might be related. Or they experience gastrointestinal problems, which can sometimes be due to inflamed intestines. Make sure the foods you are eating are not pro-inflammatory and that your so-called healthy fats—the omegas—aren't out of balance. Do your joints hurt all the time? Sugar could be to blame. Are you constantly tired or do you suffer from allergic reactions? Because food allergies can be hard to pinpoint, look at the top potential allergens in your diet, such as wheat, soy, corn, eggs, dairy, or shellfish. Cut back on consumption one food at a time to see if you can find the culprit. Keep the food out of your diet for ten days to two weeks, then slowly introduce it back in to see if it makes a difference.

Arm yourself with anti-inflammatory foods and make sure you are getting the right nutrients for your body. Some anti-inflammatory foods to include in your diet: kelp, coconut oil, extra virgin olive oil, sea vegetables, cruciferous vegetables, blueberries, turmeric, ginger, garlic, green tea, and sweet potatoes.

YOU ARE NOT GETTING ENOUGH PRIMARY FOOD

What is primary food? Primary food includes healthy relationships, physical activity, a fulfilling career—basically, anything that satisfies your hunger for life.[19] We live for experiences, for happiness, for accomplishments, for love, for family and excitement. But too often, people use secondary food (the food we ingest) to satisfy their needs for primary food, which doesn't work. Oftentimes, it's not about what we're eating or not eating; it's about everything else going on in our lives. Unhappy in your job? Your relationship? Your friendships? Perpetually stressed? All of these have an impact on how your body *reacts* to your food and your surroundings, putting unnecessary strain on your body, which can even cause illness. When not getting enough primary food, you can suffer from depression, obesity, fatigue, high blood pressure, heart disease, and more. So, examine what else is going on in your life and where you can make improvements other than in your diet.

YOU ARE ALWAYS LOOKING FOR THE QUICK FIX (I.E., DIET BOOKS)

Who dreamed up the concept of diet books? (A multi-billionaire, that's who.) If you listen to *anything* I say here, listen to this: *Stop* reading diet books. Don't follow the new trend, what worked for your friend, or what all the celebrities are doing. I repeat: *Stop reading them.*

A prime example: A man tried three completely separate diets one after the other—protein only; a "balance" of proteins, carbs, and fat; and of course, the high-carb, low-fat diet. The result? He lost the exact same amount of weight on all three diets. Why? Because he was eating *less* and moving *more*. Every time, as soon as he got off the "magic" diet, the weight came back threefold.

How many times have you heard this? Someone raves about a diet because it worked. Then they get off of that diet, and old habits return. If diets worked, everyone would be healthy, but we're not. We are medicated, sick, and beyond confused. Many of us are obese. We look to profitable companies and "experts" to tell us what to do, instead of listening to ourselves and our bodies.

While there are thousands of books, opinions, and studies "proving" that high-protein diets or low-fat diets work, or that low-carb diets are the only way to go, these diets are not the solution. They are not sustainable. I can eat 1,500 calories per day of highly processed, cheap food and not lose weight. Or I can eat 2,500 calories a day of good, healthy, whole foods and still lose weight because I'm eating more of the right foods and less of the wrong ones. It's about the quality of your food—not your caloric intake. (Of course, you need to be realistic and remember to balance your eating with your activity. You can still get too much food, even if it's the right food.)

We've become exceptionally brilliant at spouting off information we don't really understand or can back up with case study 1, 2, or 3. *Pair this "slow" carb with this "fast" carb and the weight will just fall off! Eat everything, but in moderation. Just eat small amounts. Just eat protein. Just eat healthy fats and cabbage and drink water with lemon.*

Stop listening to the noise. Instead of following diet rules and depriving yourself of the foods you love, remember that your tastes are learned. And the great thing about tastes is that, much like anything in life, they can be *un*learned. You can learn to like vegetables if you really want to. You can learn to move your body in a way that feels good to you. The benefits you reap just from making the right food and exercise choices and limiting the stressors in your life can open new doors to health and longevity.

When it comes to dieting or that quick fix, we don't think about the stress we put on our bodies. We think of losing weight as a good thing, and it can be sometimes, but nutritional stress is a very real factor in your health. If you were to pick up a nutrition science book and actually read what your body goes through just to digest a piece of fruit, it is exhausting (see page 31 for details on digestion).

Each person's body digests and processes nutrients differently. Some people perform better with coffee, and for others it's literally toxic. The same goes with grains, dairy, meat, etc. It's all specific to *your* body, *your* system, and how sluggish it has become (or how efficient). That is why it is so important to pay attention to how you feel after you eat.

Bottom line? Diets don't work. They've never worked. They are a temporary way of dealing with this great necessity of having to eat every single day. Developing a healthy relationship with food is an essential part of enjoying your life. But the word "healthy" doesn't have to mean raw veggies and sprouts. You define what a healthy diet means for you.

Top Five Common "Life" Excuses and How to Overcome Them

Start looking at all the elements in your life. Are you consistently eating on the run because you're busy? Are you too tired to cook? Do you always fall off the wagon? Look over the common excuses below and find out how to end the cycle once and for all.

Remember: You have to eat to survive, so you might as well figure out how to have a healthy, happy relationship with food.

MY JOB IS TOO STRESSFUL

A stressful job usually means long hours, running around at the mercy of everyone else, and often not giving much thought to what you're eating. While you can do great one day, you might go the next three without eating breakfast. There's no consistency, and this can spell trouble in the long run. Whether you have a desk job that requires you to sit all day, you're running all over town, or you stay at the office well past the typical nine-to-five shift, you have to find ways to sneak healthy habits into your life. Ask yourself: What is the nature of my job? Does it require sitting for long periods of time? Do I have to go out to expensive client dinners? Do I often work long hours without a break?

If so, arm yourself with the following tools:

- Set a timer to remind yourself to get up every hour. Stretch. Walk around your office or go get some water.
- Set a timer to remind yourself to have a snack or meal every three hours. Even if it's small, it's vital to keep your engine stocked.
- Stash snacks in your desk, in your car, in your gym bag, etc. Have non-perishables like energy bars, dried fruit, or nuts on hand so you can easily down a snack whenever you get the chance.
- Locate healthy restaurants or markets within close proximity to work, so if you get a few minutes, you can walk to nearby places and get orders to go.
- Find healthy spots that might deliver to your office when you just can't leave.

■ If you go out for work dinners or lunches, find out where you'll be dining and look up the menu online. Familiarizing yourself with the menu and knowing what you want will help you stay on course with your healthy goals. Often, if we have to make hurried, last-minute decisions, we'll cave and opt for the less-healthy choice.

While your job is incredibly important, eating for life is more important. Look at the priorities in your life. Where does eating healthy rank on that list? If it's not near the top, it's time to restructure a bit until you can make it a priority. By using the tools, tips, and recipes in this book, you should be able to come up with a game plan that can be implemented over the long term—not for a quick fix.

MY PARTNER DOESN'T WANT TO EAT HEALTHY

We have the best intentions in every relationship. We want to bring out the best versions of ourselves and of each other. We want to encourage, not cajole; inspire, not aggravate. But this doesn't always happen. In some relationships, two people might mutually encourage one another to become more fit and healthy, but most of the time, we enable each other with bad habits.

For instance, you might have had a set routine of getting up, working out, and making meals for yourself when you were single. But then you meet someone and go out, drink more, relax, exercise less, and the pounds creep up. Before you know it, you're ordering in pizza every Friday night, sporting a beer belly, and wondering how you got here.

SELF-ASSESSMENT: YOUR RELATIONSHIP AND YOUR HEALTH

If your relationship is contributing to bad habits, not to worry. There are several things you can do to get back on track. First, ask yourself these questions, and then evaluate your answers.

1. *Does my partner support my need to be healthy?*

2. *Is my partner physically active?*

3. *Does my partner care about what he/she eats, or what I eat?*

4. *Does my partner tease me about my weight?*

5. *Does my partner have health goals of his/her own?*

6. *Would my partner be willing to engage in physical activity or a healthier diet?*

EVALUATE YOUR ANSWERS

If your partner seems unsupportive or uninterested when it comes to your health, take an honest look at the possible reasons why and then have an open conversation about it. While it's not imperative to have the same fitness goals as your partner, supporting each other's exercise goals is important. If your partner is not physically active, perhaps they haven't found an activity they enjoy. This could be a chance to explore together to find something that you both love, or are at least willing to try. Oftentimes, we assume that our partners just aren't interested if they're not jumping at the chance to try that big quinoa salad or do yoga with us. This doesn't mean it's true. The next time you're about to hit the gym or the juice bar, invite your partner along. Or simply ask if they'd be interested in eating healthier or engaging in more exercise. Being direct works wonders.

Remember that teasing about your weight should not be tolerated. It's one thing if one or both of you is obese and words of encouragement are offered. It's quite another to make fun of someone's weight, especially in a relationship. Regardless of how uncomfortable it might be, call your partner out when this takes place, and get to the bottom of the teasing. Have you gained weight during the course of your relationship? Does your partner have "conditions" regarding your physical appearance that you weren't aware of? Be forthright about any unsavory comments so you can establish respect.

Once you answer these questions (honestly), you can figure out your next steps. If you're not with someone who is supportive, it's important to get to the bottom of why. Is there jealousy involved? A need to keep you away from your other interests? Sometimes partners can be threatened when you have a life outside of them—one in which you are sweating with other people, learning new skills, or having a good time without them. Here's an easy solution: Invite your partner along. Better yet, find an activity that you would both enjoy together.

If the problem isn't physical activity, it's usually food. It's so easy to get lazy, to order in and simply say, "I don't know how to cook for someone else" or "I can't afford lots of groceries" (though in almost all cases, cooking at home is actually the cheaper option).

Cooking together or working out together can foster closeness in almost any relationship. If this isn't really an option, don't let your partner's lack of time or motivation deter you from your health goals. If your partner is a late sleeper, and the only time you can work out is in the morning, set out your workout clothes the night before, get your playlist ready, and when the alarm goes off, don't hit snooze. Get up, get ready, grab a piece of fruit and some water, and hit the road or gym. Sweating first thing in the morning and coming back to a nutritious breakfast will make you feel accomplished before most of the population has even gotten their day started.

Sometimes, as much as we want our partners to be interested in everything we are, it just doesn't work out that way. If you love eating healthy and being active, don't give in to your partner's unhealthy lifestyle, or bash your partner because they don't have the same interests as you. But don't just assume your partner isn't interested, either—always ask and be willing to try new things, even if they fall outside of your comfort zone.

Be honest with your partner. Communicate if you feel like he or she is not being supportive. And if you find yourself in a truly destructive relationship, realize that you don't have to be in it. Relationships should be healthy and inspiring. Make sure yours fits the bill!

I BLOW IT IN SOCIAL SITUATIONS

Perhaps you have a good routine during the day or even during the week, but when you go out with friends or with your partner at night or on weekends, all bets are off. Suddenly, you can't resist those five drinks or that appetizer. You've read the tips about eating soup or a salad before your entrée, skipping the appetizers (which are often the unhealthiest items on the menu), or even asking for just a half portion of your food. Regardless, you end up going overboard and feeing guilty the next day.

If you're always on this up-and-down cycle, figure out what you crave and why. Are you really hungry when you go out? Do you just indulge because all your friends do? Will they give you a hard time if you don't? Do you use phrases like, "I can't eat that" or "I really shouldn't"? Instead, say, "I *don't* eat that." Saying "don't" shows that you have made your decision and it isn't up for debate. There's no room for negotiation. If you're focused on a goal, announce it to friends and family before you go out. Or frequent places where you won't be tempted to lose your resolve.

Remember that no one can force you to eat something you don't want to. Unfortunately, it's normal in our society to indulge in whatever we want, whenever we want. You're strange if you ask how food is prepared or ask the server to make concessions. Don't be apologetic in your approach. It's your right to know how food is prepared. If the chef isn't excited to cook for you and accommodate your special request, you are at the wrong place. Be specific about your likes and wants when it comes to ingredients, but leave the technique up to the chef. For example, if you say you don't like pastas or heavy carbs, but you love green vegetables, fresh herbs, and mushrooms, you are more likely to get items you like, and the chef will have some parameters to work within.

Be informative. The more information you can give about your dietary restrictions or what you like and don't like, the more likely it is that the kitchen will be set up for success, ensuring a better experience for you. Talk to your server. They are there to guide you. They should know every item and ingredient on the menu. But also be reasonable with your requests. Ask yourself: Does the restaurant have the product? How busy is the restaurant? The bottom line is that in many restaurants, it's not hard to get vegetables or opt for lower-fat fare. Seek out restaurants that offer fresh food.

If drinks are more of your problem, drink one glass of water to every glass of alcohol. Stick with clear liquor and no mixers, or a glass or two of red wine, which have been proven to be the healthier choices when it comes to alcohol. Put your glass down after every sip and be mindful. While we all have "those" nights out, think about your activities for tomorrow. Are you planning on exercising? Is what you're doing now going to be worth how you'll feel tomorrow? Just think it through.

HOW TO ORDER HEALTHY DISHES

When you do find yourself dining out, follow these tips.

- **Call ahead:** If you want something specific, check with the restaurant before you're seated and studying the menu, and ask what items might be compatible with your diet.

- **Alert your server to special dietary needs:** If you're sensitive to oil or salt or have any food allergies, speak up. It's always a good bet to ask the restaurant to go easy on the salt, as most dishes are heavily salted.

- **Inquire about vegetarian specials** (even if you're not a vegetarian): If there aren't specials, peruse the menu to see what vegetables come with the main dishes, so you might center your meal on some of those side dishes or grains.

- **"Supersize" your order:** Whatever entrée you order, ask if you can double the veggies.

- **When meat's on your mind:** Look for lean cuts of beef, fish specials, bison, lean ground turkey, or chicken. Inquire about the meat preparation, and see if you can get a smaller portion.

- **The backup plan:** If you don't see anything on the menu and the server isn't being overly helpful, ask if you can get a side of brown rice (or another grain) and beans. Many kitchens have these items on hand and can easily throw something together for you as a decent side dish. Pair with a large salad, and voilà: a healthy meal.

The key to healthy restaurant eating? Be patient. If you make a special request (such as a vegetable risotto or beans and rice), realize that it may take a while to prepare. Chefs want to make diners happy, but understand that the kitchen can get backed up. Don't let going out deter your healthy goals. Just have a plan in place (and a backup plan if that one fails).

I'M A BUSY PARENT

So many of us have been there. We're so exhausted from caring for a child that the idea of schlepping to the grocery store, unloading the car, and actually preparing a meal is the last thing on our minds. But you need healthy food to feel good, especially when caring for children. What are you to do?

If you can take one day per week to shop and a few hours to prep, you will be set for the entire week (maybe more). But first, you need to have a sit-down with your family to discuss likes and dislikes, and how to create an eating plan that will work for all of you. Ask your family:

- Does everyone eat the same thing?
- Are there any food restrictions or allergies you have to cater to?
- Do you generally eat the same things every week?
- What foods does your family particularly enjoy?
- What new foods might they like to try?

If everyone likes something different, it will be beyond frustrating to try to prepare four different meals. Instead, find some common ground. For example, if someone doesn't like Indian food, find out why: Is it the spices, the veggies, or the way it's prepared? Get to the bottom of the dilemma and find ways the whole family can be happy. If someone has an allergy or restriction, hunt for delicious recipes that will cater to their needs. Use the recipes in this book or find easy recipes that you know you can make, especially when you are short on time.

Next, prepare a grocery list with items you will need to buy every week. Type it up so you can print out a new copy each week and check off the items you need. Then make a menu for the week for your main meals, snacks, breakfasts, and anything else you might need. Do you have enough spices? Can you purchase certain items in bulk? Add any additional items you will need to your list. Shop online for the non-perishables to save you the extra trip.

GROCERY SHOPPING TIPS

Follow these tips for a more productive, enjoyable visit to the grocery store.

- **Shop at off times.** According to research, Wednesday morning is the best time to shop. However, visit your local market and find out when they get their shipments of produce and when the crowds are the least annoying (there's nothing worse than people who take up entire aisles with their carts and move at a snail's pace). For instance, Saturday at lunchtime is probably not a great time to shop. Find a time that is calming and can allow you to both shop and leave easily. If morning or afternoon shopping isn't possible, aim for after 7:00 p.m. Most of the work rush has left by then, allowing you to get in and out in no time. If you have no choice but to go at a busy time, get only the items you need for the next day or so, and then finish up at a less crowded time.

- **Stick to the perimeter of the store.** You've probably heard it before, but everything good for you is usually on the outer edges of the store. Stock up on fruit, veggies, and proteins, and then dip into the aisles for other staples, such as grains and legumes.

- **Make shopping enjoyable.** Grab a coffee and stroll through the aisles. Bring a shopping partner. Make it a weekly lunch date, where you eat and then shop. Or hit your local farmers' market. Paying cash, talking to the vendors, and sampling goods in the fresh air is always a better bet than ramming people's heels with your cart.

- **Never go to the store hungry.** Always eat before you shop so you won't pick up impulse purchases or rush and forget items. Go when you can concentrate on what you need without dreaming of ice cream or pizza.

- **Know when to spend and when to save.** Comparison shop in your area. Where can you get the best prices? Where can you afford to splurge a bit? Where can you save on bulk items? Make a budget and stick to it. While it's unfortunate that healthy food often costs more, that's just the backwards world we live in (try the money-saving tips in Chapter 12). Look at your other spending and see where you can cut back. Do you really need that six-dollar cab ride when you can walk? That five-dollar magazine? You'd be surprised where you can save in order to spend a tiny bit more on your health.

- **Decide how many days you are shopping for.** Some people do well shopping for the entire week, while others find that no matter how good their intentions, the food spoils. If you are the latter type, only purchase items for a few days. Use everything in your fridge (and make a soup with the excess veggies). Then, make a new list and go to the store within a few days of your last shopping trip. Know that you are going to eat out on weekends? Then try not to have too much food in the fridge. It's about being smart and knowing how you live and how you eat.

Once you've shopped, pick a night when you have help, or even one of your days off, and make big batches of food you can freeze: soups, chili, pasta sauce, energy bars, etc. By making large batches ahead of time, you can ensure you always have food on hand when you're running low on energy or time. Simply defrost what's in the freezer and dinner is served.

Another quick tip? Resurrect the slow cooker! Throw dry beans, a grain, and some veggies in the slow cooker before you leave for the day. Fill it to the top so you'll have leftovers, and when you get home, a delicious meal awaits. You can make wonderful meals for mere dollars, all by dumping ingredients into a pot.

Don't be afraid to get your kids involved as well. If they are old enough to help, introduce them to cooking, washing dishes, loading the dishwasher, and cleaning up after themselves. These "chores" can actually be fun for them and take the stress out of doing everything yourself.

MY KIDS WON'T EAT HEALTHY FOOD

It's a tricky thing, being a parent. Choosing what your child eats, when they eat it, and how often they eat it gets tough. Kids have food allergies. Kids don't like vegetables. Kids beg for chicken nuggets. Kids don't go outside. Kids play video games. Kids throw temper tantrums. Kids eat fast food. Once per day. Twice per day. They crave hamburgers. They drink sodas. They get fat. They grow into obese adults. They get sick. They die prematurely.

It is an epidemic that is completely reversible. It seems to be normal for kids to eat sugar, overly processed foods, and fast food. But, while some schools are making better efforts to overhaul cafeteria fare, it's a parent's job to introduce them to proper nutrition.

However, many parents let their child dictate meals. Have you ever heard a parent say, "Oh, Tommy will *only* eat macaroni and cheese and fish sticks. He doesn't like anything else." But, you have to ask yourself *why* he likes macaroni and cheese and fish sticks. When did he first have these foods? What foods has he been introduced to? If your child is introduced to fast food before a healthy salad, chances are the fast food will win. Kids don't just pop out of the womb saying, "Take me to McDonald's!" They are given this food by their parents.

Why do we opt for this greasy fare? Because it's cheap, fast, and easy. But healthy, balanced meals can be made in two minutes, five minutes, or even ten minutes. There's never an excuse good enough to eat fast food or just hand your child a donut or cookie because "that's what kids eat." Our nation's children are at such a disadvantage. They are more unhealthy and confused about food than ever before. We're not giving them a chance to be healthy.

You would never allow your child to sit around the dinner table smoking cigarettes and pounding shots of whiskey, right? Not only is that socially unacceptable, it would be illegal. So, why isn't there a law prohibiting the ingestion of grease-drenched, fat-laden, highly processed food that acts as a drug to your child?

In *Eat to Live*, Joel Furhman discusses this concept: "Many children eat donuts, cookies, cupcakes, and candy on a daily basis. It is difficult for parents to understand the insidious, slow destruction of their children's genetic potential and the foundation for serious illness that is being built by the consumption of these foods."[20]

In autopsies performed on children who died accidental deaths, there were fatty plaques and streaks (the beginnings of atherosclerosis) in the arteries of children and teens in the southeastern United States.[21] The *New England Journal of Medicine* discovered that more than 85 percent of adults between the ages of 21 and 39 are already showing clogged arteries.[22]

And research has shown that childhood diet has a greater impact on the prevalence of certain cancers than does a poor diet later in life.

All of this is to say: Stop going through the drive-through. Stop making excuses for not eating healthy greens, fruits, veggies, and grains. It's never too late to reshape taste buds, especially a child's. While you can't control what your child eats outside of the home, what goes on in the home is entirely up to you.

Figure out what foods your children love and start making healthier tweaks to them. Don't order off the kids' menu (ever). Let your kids eat the types of foods you eat. Let them develop their taste buds by giving them a wide array of fruits, veggies, spices, grains, seeds, nuts, and proteins.

Explain the benefits of vegetables and how they literally go to work, fighting inside of their bodies, demolishing all the bad guys. Don't try to hide veggies in meals, or tell them that if they eat their broccoli they can have dessert, making unhealthy food a reward for eating healthy food. Just make vegetables a normal part of *all* your meals. Make smoothies. Bake healthier cookies. Let them still enjoy the sweet stuff if they want it, but in a healthier way. Look at every ingredient you give your child. It's not about depriving them, but educating them.

Make it fun and informative, and they will often jump on board.

Bottom Line

No matter what life throws your way, you can overcome it with tangible solutions. Taking a few minutes to see what really hinders your daily progress is the first step; addressing the issues is the next. Taking small, incremental steps toward a healthier life is all you can do (and it can be quite fun in the process). Once you have a handle on how to tackle issues that might pop up, you can slash stress and be better equipped for healthy eating (even when your job or the kids or your partner try to derail you). Make health a priority.

QUICKEST WAY TO KILL THAT SWEET TOOTH: MAKE A HEALTHY CHOCOLATE PUDDING USING AVOCADO, HONEY, AND COCOA POWDER (SEE PAGE 231).

CHAPTER 6

Eat for Health

"I am not a vegetarian because I love animals. I'm a vegetarian because I hate plants."

—A. WHITNEY BROWN

Health has become a relative term. Today, if you hear your cousin Suzy has diabetes or heart disease, it's not such a surprise. It is not unusual to see obese people everywhere. Weight loss shows aren't shocking anymore, even when people have over 200 pounds to lose. Somewhere along the way, we've forgotten what healthy looks like, feels like, and really means.

Though health can be relative, there's a way to get it through proper nutrition. There's a way to bring foods into your daily diet that will shed unwanted pounds, boost energy, and cut health risks. "Yes, I want these things," you might say. But like so many other things in life, what does this *really* entail?

Health starts in your body and mind. Do you feel healthy, or is there much to be desired? Do you consistently promise that today is the day, and then fall off the wagon? Do you think you could be healthy if only you had the resources or time? We often cram so much in our schedules, we barely have time to brush our teeth, much less plan healthy eating.

While it seems like every single human being has a different opinion on what's healthy and what's not (and every restaurant has a vendetta against those looking to watch their waistlines), you can set yourself up for success—permanent, long-term success—a single meal at a time. Eating for health can start right now.

||||||||||||||||||||||||||||||||||||||||||||||||||||||||||||||||||||||||||||||||||||||||||||||||||||||||||||||||||||||||||||||||||||

SELF-ASSESSMENT: FIGURING OUT YOUR HEALTH

Ask yourself the following questions about your overall health, and then use the evaluation section to examine your answers.

>   1. *What does health mean to me? Be specific.*

>   2. *Where do I think I could be healthier? In my diet? Exercise? Relationships?*

>   3. *How often do I get sick? When do I get sick?*

>   4. *How many times per day do I eliminate?*

>   5. *If I examined a week of my eating, what do I think might be the biggest culprit of poor health lurking in my diet, based on what I have read so far?*

>   6. *If I looked at my diet as a whole over the last decade, have I primarily eaten the same way? Have I tried a bunch of diets? Have I shied away from variety? Where could I have improved my eating?*

>   7. *If I could make one positive long-term change, what would it be?*

||||||||||||||||||||||||||||||||||||||||||||||||||||||||||||||||||||||||||||||||||||||||||||||||||||||||||||||||||||||||||||||||||||

EVALUATE YOUR ANSWERS

First things first: Clear out all the clutter you've ever heard about health, and define it for yourself. Maybe health to you is breathing steadily while walking uphill. Maybe it means completing a marathon, never getting a cold, having healthy cholesterol, or playing with your kids for hours without needing to sit down.

Examine health in terms of different aspects of your life. What does it mean in your job, your relationship, and your physical being? Then make concrete plans for getting healthier, whether it's more sleep, less stress, less nagging, more laughing, more walking, more vegetables, or even a healthier colon (see page 99). Think in terms of what you can positively add to your life and what negative aspects you can trim.

Once you put your long-term goal(s) in writing, devise five ways to get there. Aim to help yourself toward your goals daily, weekly, and monthly, and before long, you will reach your goals and be on your way to permanent health.

||||||||||||||||||||||||||||||||||||||||||||||||||||||||||||||||||||||||||||||||||||||||||||||||||||||||||||||||||||||||||||||||||||||||||||||||||||||||||||||||

Really take the time to examine your answers to the self-assessment, and try to tackle them as you see fit in conjunction with your eating for overall success. It's important to examine all factors of your life before jumping into any lifestyle change. If you're unhappy with your body, this may feed into your relationships. If you are unhappy in your relationships, it can affect the way you eat or your body image. You can eat all the proper foods in the world, but if your personal life is making you sick, you're never going to reach the levels of health your body (and mind) intended. There is a solution to every problem. Figure out the problem first. And then start to ruminate on the solutions, using the steps in this chapter.

HEALTHY ELIMINATION

If you are irregular, constipated, or have other issues with elimination, it's time to take a closer look at your colon, as it's a huge indicator for internal health. A healthy colon eliminates waste regularly. Bowel movements should be shaped like a banana, should have no foul odor accompanying them (yes, that's right), and should float. What goes in must come out. If you only go once per day or even skip days, there are easy things you can do to help move the bad stuff along and out of your body:

- **Increase your fiber intake.** The best sources of fiber are veggies, produce, legumes, and grains.

- **Drink plenty of water.** Waste cannot move through the system without enough water.

- **Exercise.** Exercise wakes the body up and ensures all systems are working properly.

- **Cut out dairy.** Dairy can back you up and unnecessarily slow your system. Eliminate for 10 days and see if you become more regular.

- **Take probiotics or digestive enzymes.** If you've ever taken antibiotics, you might know that they knock out the good bacteria as well as the bad. It's always a safe bet to take probiotics to keep the healthy flora in the gut intact. Digestive enzymes can help you digest your food and pass it through the body in a more comfortable way, without excess gas.

Ten Steps to Eating for Health

I have broken down eating for health into ten simple, everyday steps. You can also incorporate some of the yummy recipes in Chapter 13 to meet all your healthy needs for the day. Peruse the steps and see which ones you can implement today. Make one a habit, and then add another healthy habit. It's about longevity, not quick results. Focus on what you can do today.

Study your answers from the quiz in Chapter 1 to see where you need improvement and then use them to see which of the steps below will be most helpful for you.

EAT BREAKFAST

This isn't newsworthy information. Everyone knows you should eat breakfast, but it's *what* you eat for breakfast, and when, that truly matters. Since your body fasts all night, it needs energy in the morning. If you get up and instantly go about your day, your body has nothing to pull energy from. It will start to burn muscle (not fat) just to keep you functioning properly. So, the first rule is to eat within an hour of waking.

If you don't like to eat a big meal in the morning, opt for no-bake energy bars, fruit, buckwheat pancakes, or a smoothie. Have five minutes? Make oatmeal and pile it high with healthy nuts, fruit, and seeds. Don't reach for coffee and a sugary treat at Starbucks. If you crave muffins and coffee, bake healthy muffins the night before so you can just grab and go in the morning. Use the recipes in Chapter 13 to satisfy all of your cravings and give you a healthy start to the day.

PACK SNACKS

While it might not be possible to bring your lunch to work every day, it is possible to pack snacks. Snacking has gotten a bad rap, and rightly so. The majority of our "snacks" are glorified junk food. But if you can take five minutes in the morning or the night before and pack two to three healthy snacks, you will be armed to keep your metabolism revved and your energy high. These snacks might include homemade energy bars or trail mix, fruit, nuts, seeds, a healthy sprouted sandwich, veggies and dip, dairy-free banana bread, or a green juice. Figure out what you really crave. Is it sweet? Crunchy? Salty? Try to accommodate your cravings in a more balanced way.

If you perpetually get tired in the afternoon, reach for a snack that will supply you with energy and not drain you. For example, instead of eating a cookie or muffin, opt for fresh fruit and almonds. Don't skip meals. Again, check out the recipes and see what quick options you can whip up.

SWAP YOUR GRAINS

One of the easiest ways to improve your diet is to look at what grains you're eating. Regardless of what you've read, carbohydrates aren't the enemy. Empty calories are. If you eat a bagel every morning, a sandwich at lunch, and pasta for dinner, you're eating highly processed items that will make you feel sluggish and won't aid you on your quest for health. Instead, look at the ingredients list. Choose items with the fewest ingredients and the most health benefits. Stay away from white flour, hydrogenated oils, sugar, and sodium. Whenever possible, purchase items that just have one ingredient.

Use this list as your grain bible: oats, barley, buckwheat, quinoa, millet, teff, spelt, brown rice, wild rice, amaranth, bulgur, and couscous. (If you do eat rice, pay attention to where it comes from, due to the recent discovery of high arsenic levels in certain types of rice.) If you currently eat white rice, choose brown or wild. If you eat pasta, try brown rice noodles, buckwheat soba noodles, mung bean noodles, or quinoa pasta (it tastes just as delicious, I promise). If you eat bread, look for organic, sprouted grain bread, which will give you a plethora of vitamins and minerals and tastes even heartier than its more processed counterparts.

If you get overwhelmed and don't know which new grains to try, just choose one per week. Make a huge batch of quinoa that can be eaten cold with salad or warmed up to pair with veggies and beans at night. Then, the next week, try something else. See what you like, how your body responds, and what tastes good to you.

GET A BLENDER

If you invest in one kitchen item, make it a blender. Take one to work if you can. Blending is one of the easiest ways to get all your greens and produce for the day if you can't get them from eating salads and whole veggies. Peel a bunch of bananas, store them in a Ziploc bag, and pop them in the freezer for a "creamy" smoothie base. Throw in some nondairy milk, a scoop of hemp protein powder, and then whatever fruits and veggies you want: spinach, kale, chard, collard greens, sliced apples, carrots, celery, parsley, etc. You name it, you can blend it.

Even if you don't love the taste (at first), if you can down even one green shake, you will instantly reap the benefits. It's far easier than eating a huge salad. So, drink your veggies. This is also a place to throw in nuts, seeds, a bit of cocoa or cacao for antioxidants, maca powder, chlorella, and other power foods. Blend well and drink often.

FIGURE OUT WHAT YOU'RE NOT WILLING TO DO

One of the most important keys to success is figuring out what you're *not* willing to do. As mentioned earlier, if you hate the grocery store, then it's not realistic to think you're going to go every two or three days. Instead, look up local food delivery services or opt for a personal shopper at your local supermarket. If you don't have time to cook, think about what you *do* have time for. Do you have time to blend something? Do you have time to boil water at night and make a big pot of quinoa before bed? Do you have time to make a five-minute burrito when you get home? Cooking doesn't have to be complicated. Do you hate prepping veggies? Buy them chopped instead. If you know you're not willing to give up dessert, figure out what you can't live without and learn to make it healthier (see the dessert recipes in Chapter 13 and tips for overcoming any obstacle in Chapter 12). Being realistic is one of the first steps to getting healthy. Be honest with yourself and come up with creative ways to make your life easier—not harder.

EAT THE RAINBOW

How many meals do you eat that are truly colorful? Do you have deep, vibrant shades covering your plate, or do most meals look beige? If you always buy green apples, green lettuce, or green kale, opt for deep red apples, red leaf lettuce, or purple kale—the darker, the better. Whether you focus on just one color for the week or try to pick a fruit and veggie of every color, you will be getting an array of vitamins, minerals, and antioxidants. For instance, you might think red for the week, and choose tomatoes, apples, red peppers, Swiss chard, pomegranates, raspberries, beets, etc. Always pick produce in season for the best flavor. Make it a habit to incorporate one colorful item you haven't tried before every week. Don't get stuck buying the same produce time and time again.

EAT SWEET VEGGIES

If you consistently crave sweets and fruit doesn't do the trick, opt for sweeter veggies such as beets, carrots, sweet potatoes, onions, squash, or yams. Make butternut squash or sweet potato fries. Bake some carrots or add a beet to your fresh green juice. Because veggies are full of fiber and water, many can fill you up without making you want those extra calories from sweets. In the winter, try to stick to root vegetables and thick, warm stews. In the summer, opt for massive, colorful salads and throw a grain on top for a filling meal. Experiment to see what might take the edge off that sweet tooth.

ADD MORE

As every dieter knows, focusing on what you take out is a death sentence. We've all tried this, swearing off one food or another. It is simply not the way. Instead, what can you *add*? What have you wanted to try? Coconut water? Kombucha? Chia seeds? Kimchi? Sea vegetables? Focus on one new item per week and see how you like it, how you feel, how your body responds, etc. Think about the foods you really enjoy. If you adore peanut butter (don't we all?), try almond butter. While peanuts are a legume and tote a healthy dose of protein, peanuts are also one of the dirtiest foods around and one of the top allergens. They are extremely susceptible to contaminants, especially aflatoxin, a cancerous toxin also found in meat.[23] If that doesn't deter you, this might: In every pound of peanut butter, there can be 150 bug fragments and 5 rodent hairs![24]

The fact is that a lot of our favorite foods aren't healthy and don't do us any favors. Make healthy swaps and see if you notice a difference in how you feel. If you use raw sugar, try Sucanat. If you use olive oil to cook, switch to coconut oil (yes, olive oil is still a healthy oil, but when you eat coconut oil, your body uses those fats for fuel instead of storing them in your fat cells). If you drink regular milk, try unsweetened almond. Don't cut things out—simply swap, and then add more. Look at where your diet could use some extra color, more omegas, or less sugar, and decide how you can expand your diet. Surprisingly, you might like some of these new items even more than what you're used to.

GO OUT FOR TREATS

If you know that making healthier cookies or brownies just isn't going to cut your craving, or that having sweets or salty foods around is setting you up for failure, don't keep these items in the house. Stock your fridge with healthy fare and then, when the craving strikes, make it a family affair. Go for a walk to your favorite bakery. Or drive, indulge, and then take the kids to a park to walk around or play. Plan an activity around your treat, or even seek out restaurants or grocery stores that offer vegan baked goods. (You'd be shocked at how little you can tell the difference.) Know your weaknesses, and then plan accordingly.

ADD FLAVOR

If you've eaten baked chicken breasts and steamed veggies in the past, you know that flavor can be lacking in some "health foods." When eating vegan, herbs and spices are beyond helpful in creating truly satisfying meals. Rather than purchasing dried, bottled seasonings, check your local farmers' market for fresh herbs. Try something new like garlic chives or tarragon. Fresh herbs are powerhouses of nutrients.

You need to know how to store herbs properly to get the maximum life span. You can cut the ends off of most herbs, place them in a jar of water, cover the top of the jar with a plastic bag, and store in the fridge (though certain herbs, like basil, should be kept at room temperature). You can also wrap dry herbs in a damp paper towel, place them in a Ziploc bag, and store in the fridge. Research individual herbs to see which way works best.

With these 10 simple tips, you can eat your way to health a single meal at a time. Take it slow. Choose one tip to focus on this week. Try to master it before moving on to something else. Decide which tip would be the simplest for you to implement, and try that one first. Focus on the bigger picture—long-term health.

Bottom Line

Remember to define what health means to you, and then where positive changes can be made in your daily life, first via short-term goals and then via long-term goals. Every day, ask yourself how you might be healthier, how you could think healthier, how you could act healthier. Love, laughter, and happiness are all contributors—enjoy your health and the process of getting there.

QUICKEST WAY TO EAT FOR HEALTH: MAKE A SMOOTHIE AND PACK IT WITH POWER FOODS.

CHAPTER 7

Eat for Your Age

"You've got bad eating habits if you use a grocery cart in a 7-Eleven."
—DENNIS MILLER

It will come as no surprise that we need varying nutrients and amounts of food throughout our lives. While we usually triple in size our first year and grow at a rapid pace for the first three years of our lives (and again during our teenage years), our nutritional needs change and shift into adulthood.

The amount of food we need as children differs drastically from what we need as adults, when we are over 50, and beyond. However, the vital nutrients remain the same, especially when entering a more plant-based way of living. Can you be healthy from birth without meat or dairy? Absolutely. In fact, many believe childhood is a chance to truly begin your child's life toxin-free, starting with food intake (though our polluted environment is another subject entirely).

It's up to you as a parent to expose your children to the right foods for their bodies, but this can seem like a daunting task. There are so many conflicting suggestions, requirements, and studies that it's hard to know which way to look in terms of a proper nutrition plan for a child, a teen, an adult, or a senior citizen.

While I don't have all the answers, I do know that following your intuition often goes a long way, especially in terms of healthy eating. Does it make sense to feed children candy and fast food? Is that what we're supposed to have? Common sense tells us no, though if these foods are a rarity and not an everyday staple, your child is probably fine. But giving individuals the chance to truly be healthy from the start of their lives to the end of their lives has so much to do with their own bodies' reactions to food, becoming educated about food, and a bit of experimentation. These are the best ways to ensure your health, so start young.

Since our bodies are all unique and we have varying requirements and circumstances that cause us to eat and process foods differently, use this guide to meet *basic* needs and requirements. Individualize as needed.

Infant/Toddler/Child

What you eat as a child can establish healthy habits later in life. Introducing a child to a wide variety of foods, nutrients, and minerals can set the stage for a healthier life.

If possible, breast milk is the absolute best nutrition a child can get, especially for the first six or seven months (and often much, much longer). Breast milk is a child's perfect food, specifically designed for their individual nutritional needs. The breast milk can even shift during the course of a feeding to satiate thirst (the foremilk) or give more fatty nutrients (the hindmilk). Once other foods are introduced, breast milk should still be the mainstay of an infant's diet. Offering breast milk first and then introducing other foods is easier on infants' systems and will ensure they are getting the majority of their calories from breast milk.

Whether you begin with cereals, fruits, or grains, a good tip is to go slowly and even mix a little of your breast milk with the chosen food to give the child a familiar taste. However, if using breast milk isn't possible, know that nondairy milk is never a substitute. While it can be introduced later as a supplemental dose of protein and nutrients as a child grows, it should not be the bulk of any child's diet.

Many sources suggest rice cereal should be the first food a child tries. Why? Because, universally, there are limited allergies to rice. However, don't be afraid to start with fruits and venture into vegetables, then grains, to ease their systems into healthy, fresh foods. Since fruits are full of simple sugars that often don't have to be broken down like those in complex grains, they can often be easier on a child's system.

Most vegan babies will need a bit of help in the vitamin D, vitamin B12, DHA, and even the iron departments. Discuss with your holistic practitioner or pediatrician the best plan for you and your child to supplement accordingly.

As babies grow into toddlers, appetites can become finicky but proper food intake is still key. Paying special attention to protein intake from good, quality legumes and grains is vital, as well as calcium from dark, leafy greens and soy (if no allergy presents itself) for proper bone growth. Expose children slowly to new foods and be patient. Make eating fun and not torturous. Celebrate the different colors of the rainbow. As toddlers grow up, let them get involved in preparing their own meals.

Once breast milk is no longer part of the picture, it's important to supplement accordingly with other sources. Diets can be enhanced with fortified soy milk (the highest in protein) or almond, rice, hemp, or coconut milk. While this is not a replacement for breast milk in any capacity, it's still important to get a variety of vitamins from these nondairy options. Concentrating on vitamin B12 with plant foods or a child-friendly supplement is also key, as well as DHA for brain development and iodine (easily gotten through sea vegetables).

Have a picky eater on your hands? Don't assume your child won't eat vegetables just because he refuses once or twice. It can take numerous tries until a child decides if he wants to make that food part of his life (and it might be a good idea to reintroduce it a few months down the line if he's not interested at first). Always introduce foods one at a time to give children's very delicate systems time to adjust. Also make sure to have a good rotation of foods so the child doesn't get used to, and then only want, a handful of foods.

What about so-called superfoods? Can a child have them? Yes. Superfoods, such as chlorella, spirulina, nutritional yeast, and coconut water, are safe for children and incredibly beneficial. Chlorella is a complete protein, contains all B vitamins, vitamin C, vitamin E, and major minerals. It helps immune function, improves digestion, and accelerates healing, so it's a little force field for a child's body. Spirulina has the antioxidant equivalent of seven servings of vegetables. It contains vitamin K, vitamin A, iron, and chlorophyll, which all help and protect the body. The book *Baby Greens* (see page 249) shares numerous baby-friendly recipes using these foods.

Pay special attention to:

Calcium	Vitamin B12
DHA	Vitamin D
Essential fats	Vitamin K
Iodine	
Protein	

Teen

Growing teens need just as much nutrition as infants (growing is critical at this stage), but this is a time when proper nutrition is often ignored. The stressors of school, sports, and active social lives make pizza and soda the everyday norm. Teens often forget to eat and are so busy with activities that they will just grab whatever is in sight. Teaching teens to always have healthy snacks on hand and ingest a balanced diet of healthy, natural foods is essential at this stage and can completely alter their foray into adulthood and beyond.

Focusing on protein from healthy sources such as legumes, seeds, tofu, and tempeh will help build strong, lean muscle. Getting enough water and fiber from fresh produce will flush toxins from the body and help keep the body regular. Getting enough iron (especially for menstruating girls) from dark, leafy greens, lentils, soybeans, pumpkin seeds, bran flakes, molasses, and sea vegetables will help lend energy to growing bodies. Calcium from dark, leafy greens, bean sprouts, dried fruit, beans, quinoa, chia seeds, fortified nondairy milks, yogurts, and soy products will ensure healthy bones and teeth (and will be much kinder to the body than dairy). Getting enough omegas and DHA will help brain function and focus. Loading up on vitamin D from shiitake or white mushrooms, nutritional yeast, sunshine, and sea vegetables will help the body absorb calcium.

Teaching your teen about proper food intake and supplementing accordingly when they can't get everything from their diets will make a vast difference in hormone fluctuations, mood swings, and proper growth. One of the best gifts is to teach teens how to cook and eat healthy, especially when venturing off to college, when they are often left on their own to grab unhealthy fare. If they know the benefits of healthy eating and can whip up quick five-minute meals, or know how to read nutrition information to make the best choices possible, they will be set up for permanent success.

Pay special attention to:

Calcium	Omega-3s
DHA	Protein
Fiber	Vitamin B12
Iron	Vitamin D

Adult

Being an adult is the perfect time to undo some damage from your youth and set the stage for disease prevention later in life. By protecting yourself now, you can head into the next phase of your life armed with strong bones and a healthy body. Cutting back on processed sugars, alcohol, and heavy restaurant meals and instead replacing those foods with fresh, wholesome, organic food is key. Pay close attention to the suggestions in the rest of this book, which are perfect for an adult's life. Focus on getting foods in their most natural state, taking a supplement if necessary, engaging in physical activity, and drinking plenty of purified water.

Pay special attention to:

Calcium	Potassium
Iron	Protein
Omega-3s	Vitamin B12
Phytonutrients (active compounds found in plants)	Vitamin D

Fifty Plus

So many ailments age brings can be reversed or slowed with food and proper exercise. Boosting cognitive function (via healthy fats and vegan DHA from algae), keeping bones healthy (from dark, leafy greens and soy products), and maintaining a properly functioning nervous system (with plenty of vitamin B12, sunshine, and nutritional yeast) can stave off common problems that are often misdiagnosed or treated with medication. It's also a good idea to boost intakes of critical vitamins (B, D, iron) and protein to arm your body against any impending ailments.

Pay special attention to:

Calcium

DHA

Iron

Omega-3s

Protein

Vitamin B12

Vitamin D

From birth to death, we need so many of the same nutrients (though at some stages—infancy, teen, and 50 plus—these nutrients become increasingly more important for health and longevity than at others). But the critical nutrients are easy to get if you know where to look, and they can make all the difference between sickness and health.

Menus for Life

Regardless of your dietary restrictions or preferences, there are ways to get everything you need from a plant-based diet. So what would a typical "perfect" vegan day look like in the teen-to-adult world (with amounts varying according to activity levels)? I'm going to give you three different options: soy free, nut free, and gluten free, since so many individuals have allergies or prefer different menus.

Experiment with one of the daily menus below and see how your energy soars and how much better you feel. (For more menu ideas, see page 242.)

Soy-Free Vegan

MEAL ONE

- 1 cup (234 g) cooked steel-cut oats topped with chia seeds, blueberries, blackstrap molasses, and walnuts
- 1 cup (237 mL) fortified nondairy milk (almond, rice, hemp, or coconut)

What's in a meal: complex carbs, protein, and fiber from oats; Omega-3s, protein, calcium, and fiber from chia seeds; antioxidants from blueberries; iron from molasses; Omega-3s from walnuts; calcium, protein, and vitamins D and E from nondairy milk

MEAL TWO

- Green juice

What's in a meal: antioxidants, fiber, calcium, beta-carotene, and vitamin C

MEAL THREE

- 2 slices sprouted bread
- 1 large bowl lentil soup
- Kale and collard greens cooked in coconut milk with 1 teaspoon coconut aminos

What's in a meal: fiber, protein, and complex carbs from bread; protein and iron from lentils; fiber, folate, calcium, iron, and zinc from veggies; magnesium, phosphorous, vitamin B, and potassium from coconut milk; amino acids and protein from coconut aminos

MEAL FOUR

- Sprouted hummus
- Veggie sticks
- ½ cup (72 g) sprouted trail mix

What's in a meal: protein and fiber from sprouted hummus; fiber and phytonutrients from veggies; amino acids, essential fats, and protein from trail mix

MEAL FIVE

- 1 cup (234 g) teff
- 1 cup (about 177 g) legumes
- 1 cup (about 180 g) steamed or sautéed greens with coconut oil and sea vegetables
- 2 tablespoons nutritional yeast

What's in a meal: protein and fiber from teff; protein from legumes; phytonutrients from sautéed greens; healthy fats from coconut oil; iodine, iron, vitamin B12, and calcium from sea vegetables; vitamin B12 from nutritional yeast

Gluten-Free Vegan

MEAL ONE

- Vegan shake made with hemp protein, soy yogurt, frozen fruit, and cacao powder

What's in a meal: complete protein and omegas from hemp protein; probiotics, protein, vitamin D, and calcium from soy yogurt; antioxidants and protein from frozen fruit and cacao

MEAL TWO

- Buckwheat pancakes topped with fresh nuts and berries

What's in a meal: iron, fiber, zinc, and protein from buckwheat; essential fats from nuts; antioxidants from berries

MEAL THREE

- Tofu sandwich wrapped in butter lettuce topped with sprouted hummus, avocado, and tomato

What's in a meal: complete protein, calcium, and fiber from tofu; fiber and protein from sprouted hummus; phytonutrients, essential fats, and lycopene from toppings

MEAL FOUR

- 1 cup (190 g) cooked brown rice
- 2 cups (260 g) dinosaur kale with sesame oil and chia seeds

What's in a meal: complex carbs, iron, and fiber from brown rice; iron, calcium, and folate from kale; essential fats from sesame oil; omegas, protein, and fiber from chia seeds

MEAL FIVE

- Black bean burger
- Sweet Potato Fries (see page 215) topped with pumpkin seeds
- Side salad

What's in a meal: complex carbs, fiber and, protein from black bean burger; antioxidants and vitamins from sweet potato fries; iron from pumpkin seeds; phytonutrients from side salad

Nut-Free Vegan

MEAL ONE

- Apricot and hemp milk muesli (modify recipe on page 221)

What's in a meal: calcium and iron from apricots; vitamin D, omegas, and protein from hemp milk; complex carbs and fiber from oats

MEAL TWO

- Green smoothie made with hemp seeds, spinach, nondairy milk, spirulina, chlorella, and cacao powder

What's in a meal: phytonutrients from greens; omegas and protein from hemp seeds; iron from spinach, complete protein and calcium from nondairy milk; vitamin A from spirulina; phytonutrients from chlorella; antioxidants from cacao powder

MEAL THREE

- Tomato soup
- Grilled "cheese" (Daiya cheese alternative and nutritional yeast on sprouted bread)

What's in a meal: lycopene from tomatoes; complex carbs and fiber from sprouted bread; vitamin B12 from nutritional yeast

MEAL FOUR

- Celery sticks
- Sunflower seed butter
- Raisins

What's in a meal: fiber from celery; omegas from sunflower seed butter; antioxidants and iron from raisins

MEAL FIVE

- Asian stir-fry with tempeh, Bragg's Liquid Aminos, veggies, dulse, and barley

What's in a meal: complete protein from tempeh; amino acids from Bragg's Liquid Aminos; phytonutrients from veggies; complex carbs and fiber from barley; vitamin B12 and iodine from dulse

Bottom Line

No matter what meals you eat in a day, supplement accordingly (especially if you're a plant eater) and pay attention to specific needs for your age, your lifestyle, your activity level, the nature of your job, the stressors in your life, etc. Try to put it all together to fuel your body in a way that is conducive to your lifestyle.

Get your family on board and make meals that will cover a wide array of nutrients in every bite. Have fun with your food, and know that every smart choice you make is an insurance policy for your health.

QUICKEST WAY TO BOOST ENERGY: GET A GOOD DOSE OF VITAMIN B12.

CHAPTER 8

Eat for Fitness

"I've been on a diet for two weeks and all I've lost is two weeks."
—TOTIE FIELDS

Whether you are just starting an exercise program or are used to working out and enjoy being fit, the eating techniques that elite athletes use to stay in peak shape are more accessible to you than you'd think. There's no big secret to eating for fitness. It's simply in the execution: eating in a way that complements your individual level of activity, whatever that may be. And even the "healthiest" among us—athletes and the very physically fit—aren't always eating the right things, or eating them at the right times.

So no matter what your individual fitness level, knowing the right way to work out and how to fuel your workouts is key. Understanding how much food you need and for what activities is vital to getting the physique you want while reaching optimal health so you stay ailment free in the future.

It's important to know that even if you're fit, you can negate your daily activities with food intake alone. Most people grossly overestimate what they burn during a typical 45-minute or hour-long sweat session, and can ruin all of that hard work with just a sugary coffee drink.

Over the years as a trainer and nutrition consultant, "What should I eat before and after exercise?" is one of the most common questions I'm asked. But if you ask five different trainers, fitness professionals, or even doctors, you will most likely get five completely different answers. Eat complex carbs. Eat simple carbs. Eat protein. Eat fat. But what's the best bet for *your* body?

Eating for fitness requires an individual look at what your goals are, what you're currently doing, and what your specific physical needs might be. For instance, if you are training for a marathon, your nutritional needs will differ drastically from those of a bodybuilder. While the foundation is the same, the ratios are different. An endurance athlete needs more calories and carbohydrates so they don't use up all of their glycogen stores with activity. Bodybuilders, on the other hand, tend to slash carbohydrates and load up on protein to build muscle.

While these are opposite ends of the spectrum, you probably fall somewhere in the middle, and can reach a point where you don't have to pay too much attention to the ratios. Instead, focus on eating well-balanced meals catered to your training regimen and recovery.

SELF-ASSESSMENT: FOOD AND FITNESS

Take a few minutes and answer these questions to gauge where you are with your workouts and your eating and where you could use improvement.

1. *What is my current fitness regimen?*
2. *How would I like to improve it?*
3. *How many times per day do I currently eat? Are those meals evenly spaced, or are there large gaps between meals?*
4. *Where could I improve my pre- and post-workout nutrition?*
5. *What seems to be my biggest downfall when it comes to fitness?*
6. *If I have a carb-heavy meal, do I get tired after?*
7. *How much protein do I eat? Do I feel sluggish after I eat a lot of protein?*
8. *Do I feel properly fueled before and after my workouts?*
9. *Am I seeing results with my fitness routine, or have I reached a plateau?*
10. *What's harder—pushing myself during my workouts, or eating clean (i.e., healthy grains, seeds, legumes, and produce)?*

EVALUATE YOUR ANSWERS

Be honest about your fitness regimen in relation to your dietary needs. Often, we drastically overestimate the number of calories we need. Write down your fitness routine for an entire week: the number of reps, sets, and hours you exercise. Then compare this to your food intake and use the exercises in this book and the tips in Chapter 10 to create a routine that works for you.

If you are in the mindset of protein, protein, protein, your body could be overtaxed by having to consistently break down meat (or if you're a vegan, fake meats or too many beans and legumes). Try cutting back slightly if you are a protein "overeater," and see if your energy and strength levels stay intact. See Chapter 3 for more on protein.

Identifying where you could use some help with fitness is key to meeting your goals. If you can hammer out a hard workout but fall into a bowl of chips and guacamole when Friday night rolls around, then diet is obviously your focus. But if you eat well and just can't find the motivation you need to make proper fitness gains, enlist the help of friends or a professional. There are always ways to meet your goals, regardless of your issue.

Principles of Eating for Fitness

Once you have a firm grasp on your fitness and nutrition needs, try to incorporate the following principles into your daily life.

EAT THE RIGHT FOODS PRE AND POST WORKOUT

The first step to eating for fitness? Paying attention to what you eat pre and post workout. This doesn't mean exercising on an empty stomach and then eating a protein-heavy shake or sugary sports drink, which has become the norm. What you eat before, and especially after, your workouts can make or break your energy level for the entire day and have a drastic effect on your fitness level. If you burden your body with too much protein or carbs before or after you workout, your body will use the energy it needs for exercise and recovery on trying to break down your food instead. With a few simple switches, you can reap the benefits of maximizing your workout potential—all by changing what you eat before and after the gym.

PRE-WORKOUT FUEL

The key is to find something to eat before you work out that will immediately be used as fuel. Simple carbohydrates are the preferable choice, so your body doesn't have to use complex carbs, or convert complex carbs to simple carbs because it runs out of energy.

What does this mean? Simple carbohydrates, also called simple sugars, are those that don't have to be broken down. They are there to be used for energy—preferably immediately. But remember there's a difference between table sugar and the naturally occurring sugars found in fruit (which is the type of simple sugar you are aiming for). Complex carbohydrates, or starches, are made up of three or more sugars and must be broken down before they can be used. Complex carbs are found in foods like pasta, oats, bread, certain vegetables, and legumes. They take the longest to digest.

If you eat a high-fiber cereal pre workout (complex carbs) or have a piece of toast (complex carbs) with peanut butter, your body has to use its energy to digest that food (i.e., to break down those complex grains and fat), instead of supplying your muscles with immediate fuel. A lot of times, people "gas out" in their workouts before they should because their bodies are using energy to digest food instead of fueling their exercise.

The best pre-workout foods are ones that are easily digestible. Fruit is the optimal choice, with dates being one of the best fruits because they are rich in glucose and they are used for immediate energy. The body (the liver, specifically) doesn't have to convert them to a different form of fuel to use them. They are there and ready to go. Can't stomach dates first thing in the morning? Try a grapefruit, apricots, raisins, or a banana.

If you're going for a longer, more intense workout, one of the best pre-workout snacks, adapted from Brendan Brazier's book *Thrive*, is the following:

Energy Bites[25]

>   5 dates
>   2 tablespoons coconut oil
>   2 teaspoons lemon zest
>   1 teaspoon lemon juice

Blend all ingredients in a food processor or blender. Shape into small, portable balls.

- -

Why coconut oil, you might ask? Isn't that laden with fat? Won't your body have to convert it to something else to use for energy? Or won't it just be stored as fat (since you might already know that fat is the last thing we burn)?

As discussed in Chapter 2, coconut oil actually isn't stored as fat in the body. Because it is a medium-chain triglyceride, our bodies prefer to use it as energy instead of storing it as fat. This makes it one of the best power foods around. In the fuel bites above, the quick energy from the dates combined with the good fats from the coconut oil will keep you sustained for hours.

Keep in mind that these fuel bites are optimal before intense exercise (this doesn't mean a 20-minute walk around the block). Also pay attention to what you're eating the night before. Often, what you ingest the evening prior is vital to optimum performance the next day. If you eat a bunch of sugar or a heavy meal, it's hard for your body to have the quick energy it needs to perform. Poor evening eating can lead to early-morning fatigue and reduced workouts, even if you're doing something low impact.

POST-WORKOUT FUEL

Obviously, what you eat after your work out is most important, since the body needs the proper fuel to recover. Post workout is *all* about recovery.

You may have been taught to down a protein shake within an hour, because it replenishes muscle. But after exercise, your body is tired. It needs simple sugars and a little bit of protein to instantly get to work. If you pump your body full of heavy protein, fat, and complex carbs—found in a lot of popular protein shakes—it has to work extra hard to digest them. You've already exhausted your body from working out, so if it's working to digest the shake, it has no energy for repairs. Your body can't digest your food and repair itself at the same time. You need to give it instant energy instead.

Many ingredients found in some of the most popular protein shake brands are highly processed and laden with chemicals. Not only that, but when you down a shake with a lot of protein immediately after a tough workout, all the blood rushes to the stomach for digestion instead of to the extremities to help repair muscles. A quick recovery drink or a shake made mostly of simple carbs are better choices.

A recovery drink could consist of some variation of the following: water, a banana, blueberries, ground flax, and two tablespoons hemp protein, all blended to give you immediate fuel. Then, in an hour, you can have your more protein-based shake (my personal favorite is Vega One—it has everything you could ever need in a protein powder, including superfoods like maca, chlorella, and sacha inchi seeds, and will reduce soreness completely) or a nutrient-rich, balanced meal. Check out other brands like Garden of Life RAW Protein as well to see what works best for your dietary needs.

So, to reiterate: Eat simple carbs before and immediately after your workout (along with a bit of protein post workout), and then a nutrient-rich meal an hour after your recovery drink. Learning the science of your body can completely change your ability to recover from your workouts, as long as you are eating the proper fuel.

A few things to remember if you're still eating a traditional American diet:

- You might want to skip the dairy in your pre-workout meal. Milk often feels "sour" in the stomach when you exercise because it is hard to digest.
- Avoid very acidic juices before your workout and processed, sugary drinks after.
- Don't go overboard on the fat you ingest before a workout, as it's the last thing you burn off. (As mentioned earlier, coconut oil is an exception to this rule.)
- Pay attention to portion size. Eat according to your activity level. There's a large difference between the needs of a cyclist going 50 miles and those of someone who is just going to the gym to lift weights or do a quick cardio session. Supply yourself with enough to fuel your body, but don't go overboard.
- Eat 40 minutes to an hour before your workout and within one hour of completing your workout.
- Cardinal rule? Always eat before and after!

SWAP YOUR PROTEINS

As you know, we are a nation obsessed with protein. We often think that being fit is synonymous with eating enough protein, but in fact, our ratios are way off. You actually only need around 10 to 15 percent of your diet to be protein for maximum health, even if you exercise often. If you're trying to put on a ton of muscle, you may want to boost your intake of plant-based proteins or vegan protein powders, but a little goes a long way. You can continue to put on muscle with a wide array of foods, not just protein. So, if you are an egg-, whey protein-, chicken breast-, turkey-, tuna-, and bison-loving individual (as I used to be)—in other words, if your meals are focused around your protein—it's time to make your life a lot easier, healthier, and cheaper. Choose from the following plant protein sources: hemp, legumes, pseudograins, seeds, tofu, or tempeh (unless you have an aversion to soy). Consult Chapter 3 for in-depth information on managing your protein intake. Make small changes and see how you feel.

EAT HIGH-ENERGY MEALS

If you're someone who mindlessly eats, then it might be a good idea to plan your meals, even if only for a day. When you're rushed and hungry, it's easy to reach for quick food, and things can end up out of balance, even if those foods seem healthy. Instead of reaching for one of the many protein bars lining the shelves, make your own. Drink smoothies. Pump your body full of high-fuel snacks and meals, so you don't have to rely on overly processed foods or caffeine for an instant boost.

A sample healthy day could look like the following:

MEAL ONE (PRE WORKOUT)

- Dates or banana

MEAL TWO (POST WORKOUT)

- Recovery shake: 1 scoop hemp protein, ½ cup (about 73 g) fruit, nondairy milk or water, and ice

MEAL THREE (AN HOUR LATER)

- ½ cup (117 g) steel-cut or old-fashioned oats topped with blueberries, walnuts, hemp seeds, and agave nectar or raw honey

MEAL FOUR

- Large green salad topped with broccoli, carrots, celery, peppers, avocado, cucumber, chia seeds, nutritional yeast, ½ cup (86 g) black beans, and ½ cup (about 93 g) quinoa, brown rice, teff, or millet (or whatever veggies you prefer—don't be afraid to experiment to see what you like)

MEAL FIVE

- Green Superfood Energy Bar (see page 233)

MEAL SIX

- Sweet potato, millet, or quinoa
- Veggies or salad and sea vegetables
- Legumes

MEAL SEVEN (OPTIONAL)

- Chocolate Ice Cream (see page 230) or Chocolate Pumpkin Pudding (see page 231)

Attempt to plan your meals for a day and see if you can stick to the general game plan. If it's too hard, examine where you had issues and see how you can combat them with easy recipes or good takeout options.

CHECK YOUR OMEGA RATIO

You probably know about the importance of getting your omegas, but if you are getting too many Omega-6s in relation to your Omega-3s, you could be suffering from inflammation (see page 83). This can especially hinder you in your fitness routine by causing joint inflammation and soreness. If your joints often ache and you are consistently sore despite having a healthy diet, enough rest, and enough recovery, you may want to check your omega ratios.

Getting enough Omega-3s is vital to fighting inflammation in your body, but people often tout the benefits of fish oil above all others. If you currently take a fish supplement, give your pocketbook a rest and look for a vegan omega supplement. One step better? Get all the omegas you need from hemp, chia, sacha inchi, or flax seeds. A little sprinkle on your morning oatmeal goes a long way and is easily digested. The best part? Their ratios are already intact, so you don't have to worry about the proper balance. Simply pay attention to other, outside sources of too many Omega-6s, such as canola oil, sunflower seeds, sunflower butter, safflower oil, grapeseed oil, corn oil, walnut oil, soybean oil, and even wheat.

CUT BACK ON PROCESSED SUGAR

Sugar is the devil—no, really, it is. It leads to diabetes, disease, cancer, obesity, mood swings, and a host of other health problems. Processed sugar—the real culprit—is refined sugar added to foods for sweetness and flavor. Cereals, muffins, juices, cookies, and even bread are dosed up with sugar, which is unnecessary and addictive. A 2009 study found that the average American consumed 22 teaspoons per day of added sugar, with teens coming in at 34.[26] That's way too much. While not all sugar is created equal, processed sugar will wreak havoc on your body, your pancreas, and your insulin production. It can lead to mood swings, fatigue, depression, weight gain, and even diabetes.

Not all sugar is bad, however. Sugar from fresh fruit is packed with vital nutrients, not to mention the ability to quell a sweet tooth. Many believe that to reach optimal health, you should always eat fruit on an empty stomach, and never after a meal, since the acids may mix with your food and actually putrefy your meal.

Diabetes and health risks aside, there is a direct correlation between mood and sugar intake. Children are a prime example. Ever see a child on a full-out sugar high? What about when that child comes off the sugar high? Even parents cower from the mood swing that comes with that inevitable sugar crash. Now just imagine what's happening *internally*. Sugar is dangerous for everyone—period.

Ever suffer from joint pain? Swollen eyes? Exhaustion? Irritability? Sugar could be to blame. And if your goal is increased fitness, this excess sugar will only hinder you, not help. Sugar and exercise don't mix. Joint inflammation, soreness, and decreased energy are just a few of the side effects often experienced when you mix processed sugar and exercise.

The problem with sugar is that once you get a taste for it, it's hard to break. But, you can break it without depriving yourself. Look at your diet. Where do you get added sugar? If you "need" that sweetness (and I can promise you don't—it's a learned taste and it can just as easily be unlearned), look for raw agave, raw honey, coconut palm sugar, or even Sucanat (natural cane sugar). Blend up dates to make date sugar. Or better yet, start weaning yourself off. Sugar, like cheese, is addictive. If you cut back and then reintroduce it, you will notice how awful you feel. So, if a piece of fruit doesn't cut it, opt for one of the sweet, healthy snacks or desserts in Chapter 13. Remember that one of the main principles of power eating is to figure out what you most love and learn to make it better.

Bottom Line

Try to incorporate these five tips into your daily life. As your training changes, you must change your eating as well. Don't focus on calorie counting or complicated fat and protein ratios. Instead, think about what your body actually *needs*. Have you had four servings of fruit today, but not veggies? Make a green juice or big salad to balance it out. Have you had any healthy grains? Seeds? Good sources of vegan protein (no fake meat allowed)? Make a mental checklist and plan each day in relation to your activity level.

Remember that your eating should differ daily based on your activities. And remember to always pay attention to how you feel *after* you eat. It will tell you everything you need to know.

QUICKEST WAY TO ADD INSTANT ENERGY BEFORE OR AFTER A WORKOUT: EAT DATES.

CHAPTER 9

Eat Like an Athlete

"So many people spend their health gaining wealth, and then have to spend their wealth to regain their health."

—A.J. REB MATERI

Perhaps by now you have a good idea of what health means for you, or you've reached your own personal level of fitness. Perhaps you even run races, have a great physique, or are the go-to person for your friends when it comes to nutrition and exercise. Whether this is you, or just a dream version of you, all of our diets could use improvement, especially when you are on a slightly more elite level in terms of wanting to take your nutrition to its peak. And even if you aren't an athlete, knowing how to eat like one can provide principles you can apply at any level of fitness—and it can be simpler than you think.

So what if you want to take your nutrition to the next level for performance? Many athletes wouldn't dream of cutting meat or dairy, especially endurance athletes who need copious amounts of calories to burn through. But, as the success of acclaimed vegan ultramarathoner Scott Jurek proves, it's easy to get enough calories as a vegan athlete if you know how to eat, what to eat, and when to eat. Nutrition is just as important as athletic performance, if not more important.

You might have heard that many of your favorite Olympic athletes eat plant-based diets. MMA fighters, boxers, tennis players, wrestlers, football players, golfers, runners—you name it, there are plant-based athletes to be found. To name a few:

- Brendan Brazier, professional Ironman triathlete and author of *Thrive*
- Andreas Cahling, Swedish champion bodybuilder and Olympic gold medalist in the ski jump
- Chris Campbell, Olympic wrestling champion
- Ruth Heidrich, six-time Ironwoman triathlete and USA track and field Master's champion
- Keith Holmes, world-champion middleweight boxer
- Desmond Howard, professional football star and Heisman Trophy winner
- Scott Jurek, ultramarathoner
- Georges Laraque, retired professional hockey player
- Bill Manetti, powerlifting champion
- Martina Navratilova, champion tennis player
- Paavo Nurmi, long-distance runner, winner of 9 Olympic medals and 20 world records
- Bill Pearl, four-time Mr. Universe
- Stan Price, world weightlifting record holder for the bench press
- Dave Scott, six-time winner of the Ironman triathlon
- Art Still, former Buffalo Bills and Kansas City Chiefs MVP defensive end
- Venus and Serena Williams, tennis champions
- Charlene Wong, Olympic champion figure skater

How are these athletes so successful? They know that eating plant-based diets stokes their bodies for prolonged activity. Many athletes experience eating and recovering as our ancestors once did. Their bodies are their tools, their weapons. If they don't take care of them, they will gas out. The demands on athletes are different than those on the everyday person: constant training, fueling, assessing, recovering, and making adjustments. But even if you're not an athlete, you can take advice from the way they live and train. Always look for ways to shift your eating habits, training, or even the way you live. Be receptive to changes in order to make gains. Don't stay comfortable in your routine. Pay attention to how you feel.

SELF-ASSESSMENT: TAKING YOUR FITNESS TO THE NEXT LEVEL

If you are fit, healthy, and ready to take it to the next level, whether in your training or your diet, ask yourself the following questions. Study your answers. Where do you need improvement? Then use the tips in this chapter to help you with the issues you have identified.

1. *How often do I train?*

2. *What do I eat pre and post workout?*

3. *Where could my diet use improvement?*

4. *Do I get sore?*

5. *Do I get tired post workout? If so, is it before or after I eat my post-workout meal?*

6. *How long does it take for me to recover from workouts?*

7. *Do I get cravings? If so, for what? And when?*

8. *What have I been told to eat for protein, and why?*

9. *Have I experimented with plant-based proteins versus traditional animal proteins? Which makes me feel better?*

10. *How much water do I drink per day?*

11. *What are my main sources of electrolytes?*

12. *What supplements am I taking? Do I notice a difference in supplements derived from whole foods versus popular synthetic varieties?*

EVALUATE YOUR ANSWERS

If you are an athlete, when it comes to diets, you've probably heard it all. In diets from Paleo to Atkins and beyond, protein is usually recommended as the primary source for building muscle. Think about what you've been told about protein and what you incorporate into your daily life. Does what you eat make you feel good, or have you never tried anything new? Do your research about different proteins you might be interested in and start making healthy swaps with more plant-based proteins to see how much more energy you have, how much easier they are to digest, and how they can build just as much muscle as meat. See Chapter 3 to read more about protein.

If you are a meat eater, try swapping your main protein at each meal with a plant-based protein, such as legumes, seeds, tofu, tempeh, a pea-brown rice-hemp protein blend, or even a meat substitute. See how your training goes and how your muscles feel. Then go back to meat. Which serves you better? Which gives you more energy and slashes soreness?

If hydration is an issue, remember that water flushes toxins from your body and keeps everything working properly. If you are working out for over an hour at an intense pace, consider supplementing with electrolytes to ensure you are replacing salt lost through sweat. Coconut water or a homemade recovery drink are better bets than Gatorade or other sports drinks on the market. Think simple. This goes for supplementation as well.

How to Eat Like an Athlete

While there's no canned program for eating like an athlete, there are certain guidelines to follow that can benefit anyone leading an active lifestyle. Taking cues from some of the top athletes and plant-based eaters in the world, here are my top suggestions.

CREATE YOUR OWN RECOVERY DRINK

Getting stronger is often about what you do *after* you work out, as well as during. This is also when you repair damaged tissues. Are you resting? Are you active? What are you eating? What are you replenishing with? What's your plan of attack the next day? Approach your body as you would a project or deadline. Make a plan and adhere to it.

An important part of your post-workout plan should be a recovery drink. However, sports drinks are expensive and often packed with unhealthy chemicals and sugar. According to Brendan Brazier, the leading expert on vegan sports nutrition, it's vital you get the proper nutrients and hydration pre and post workout. So instead of reaching for an expensive processed drink, create your own. Try Brendan's adapted recipe before, during, or after exercise. Just blend all ingredients and drink.

Recovery Drink[27]

Juice of ½ organic lemon

Juice of ¼ organic lime

4 Medjool dates, pitted

2 tablespoons wild-harvested honey or agave nectar

1 tablespoon hemp protein powder

1 tablespoon dulse flakes

1 teaspoon hemp oil

½ teaspoon lemon zest

1 tablespoon virgin, expeller-pressed coconut oil (optional)

½ teaspoon maca powder (optional, for extra adrenal nourishment)

You can also experiment by using coconut water as a base. Try adding different superfoods to see what boosts your performance and aids recovery.

PAY ATTENTION TO RATIOS

While this book is not about carb, protein, or fat ratios, it is important to pay attention to ratios in terms of seeds, nuts, grains, fruits, veggies, and legumes. Now that you are a more advanced power eater, where are you lacking? Are you getting too many nuts? Do you feel as good when you eat a handful of cashews as you do with almonds? Have you tried soaking seeds and nuts to unlock their true nutrient potential (see page 58)? Are you getting a wide variety of greens that supply you with all your vitamins and minerals, or do you need an additional plant-based supplement, such as chlorella, to help fill in the gaps?

Are you getting good legumes every day? Vitamin B12? Electrolytes? Where is your protein coming from? *When* are you eating that protein? How many grains are you getting per day? When do you eat them? When do you notice yourself feeling strongest? Weakest?

Start tuning in to how you feel, especially in relation to food and exercise. Make small tweaks where necessary, and don't be afraid to experiment with different types of foods and recipes to suit your particular lifestyle and daily needs.

EAT FREQUENTLY

While this is not a revelation by any means, it is vital to enhanced performance. You can't get stronger by eating just three times per day. Aim for smaller, more frequent meals, as often as you need them. If you're hungry, you need more nutrient-dense foods. If you're burning an exorbitant number of calories, add more calorie-dense foods, such as nut butters and heartier grains and legumes, to your daily eating. Pay attention to how you feel and make changes from there.

EAT FOR POWER

Power is the name of the game. Everything you eat should aid your performance. Why are you eating those seeds? That piece of fruit? That burrito? Think of your body as a furnace. What can you burn and use for fuel? What is going to repair your muscles even as you sit and do nothing? What is going to hinder your performance (too much alcohol, processed sugars, or dinners out)? You do push-ups to strengthen your upper body or run to enhance your aerobic threshold, so think of eating in the same way—it's for specific purposes and benefits. It's not to comfort or indulge (though the occasional indulgence is our given right), but to aid, strengthen, repair, extend our lives, and improve performance.

EAT FOR YOUR SPECIFIC NEEDS

While it's great to read about other athletes and what they do, or even to hear about what your teammates or workout partners might do, that doesn't matter. Your nutrition is specific for *your* body—period. What works for you doesn't work for anyone else, so you must master your own perfect eating plan. Lay out your training for an entire week. Do your days differ drastically? Do your physical or nutritional needs differ even more? Just because Joe Schmo is drinking a heavy protein shake after each workout doesn't mean you need to. You are smart. Your body is even smarter. Experiment to see what it needs and when it needs it. You will know you are eating properly when you feel great and don't suffer from energy slumps or exhaustion (unless you are severely lacking in sleep, stressed, or are unhappy in your relationships, which are all vital components to any health regimen).

Best Power Foods for Athletes

Even though you are your own individual, there are certain foods that will enhance anyone's performance and health. In terms of athletic endeavors, what are the power foods athletes most often reach for? Below are some of the best tried-and-true foods. You can try one per week and see how you like it, or add them all gradually: into smoothies, on top of salads, or in stir-fries. Or, if you'd rather get the most of these goodies in one quick drink, you can even shop Vega (myvega.com) or Garden of Life RAW Protein products, vegan protein powders that contain some or all of the ingredients below and will help take your fitness to the next level entirely.

Chia: An Aztec power food, these seeds are a great source of dietary fiber, protein, and omegas. Completely gluten-free and vegan, these little powerhouses tote more antioxidants than flax and will supply you with long-lasting energy for any of your physical activity needs.

Chlorella: Chlorella is known as a "perfect" whole food. It's a complete protein and contains all B vitamins, vitamin C, vitamin E, and major minerals. It helps immune function, improves digestion, detoxifies the body, accelerates healing, protects against radiation, relieves arthritis . . . the list goes on. It is a superfood and can be added to shakes or mixed with water and taken plain.

Coconut water: Coconut water is chock-full of electrolytes, supplying proper hydration for athletes who don't want to reach for a sugary Gatorade. Pure coconut water is the liquid found in young coconuts. Naturally fat free, low in sodium, and high in potassium, this is a good alternative if you need something slightly more hydrating than water. Read the ingredients of store-bought varieties or even opt to make your own at home!

Maca: Maca root is an Incan superfood and is sometimes thought to be an aphrodisiac. It has been known to enhance energy and stamina, and helps with fertility. It can also help with fatigue or sexual dysfunction. In powder form, you can add to smoothies or shakes.

Sacha inchi: One of the most powerful anti-inflammatory foods around, this seed (also known as the Incan peanut) is high in omegas, promotes heart health, improves mood, promotes healthier skin and vision, and helps stabilize glucose levels. It contains the highest levels of Omega-3s of any plant-based food and totes nine grams of complete protein per serving.

Sea vegetables: Sea vegetables are a wonderful source of calcium, iron, and iodine. They contain all the minerals from the ocean as well as numerous vitamins, making them one of the most nutrient-dense foods in the world.

Yerba mate: Traditionally used in various South American cultures, this tea is a perfect alternative to coffee and contains just 20 mg of caffeine per cup. When it is taken before exercise, many athletes notice enhanced performance.

When purchasing any of these foods, always search for the best-quality ingredients. Don't always jump for the sale—when it comes to high-quality foods, if it seems too good to be true, then it probably is. Research brands and items that have the purest ingredients possible. It makes a drastic difference when aiding performance.

Aim for sports-specific foods, and always fuel yourself around your activity for the best results possible.

Bottom Line

Even if you're not training for a sport or a race, you can still benefit from eating like an athlete, especially when it comes to the foods described in this chapter. Incorporate one a week into your meals to see if you notice a boost in energy, endurance, or recovery after workouts.

Don't be afraid to increase your activity level—just be sure to have an eating plan in place that supports your active lifestyle. Focus on your nutritional needs. While you can take training cues or dietary advice from your favorite athletes, remember all our bodies are different, so it's vital to tune in to your body on a daily basis to see what it might need.

QUICKEST WAY TO SPEED RECOVERY: ADD SEA VEGETABLES TO YOUR DIET.

CHAPTER 10

Work It Out

"Whenever I feel the need to exercise, I lie down until it goes away."
—ROBERT MAYNARD HUTCHINS

While we all need food to exist, most of us don't think of exercise as a necessity. But just as healthy food is important, so are a healthy mind and body. Combining the right form of movement for your body with proper eating sets the stage for internal and external health.

For me, exercise has always been a natural part of my life. When I was a kid, workout clothes were more inviting than regular clothes (as they still are to this day), and throwing my hair into a ponytail was my style of choice. Shoving headphones on and moving my body always inspired creativity in other areas of my life. Without movement, I became stagnant. Without consistently elevating my mind and pushing past uncomfortable body limits, I felt stunted somehow.

As an added bonus, my parents were always at the YMCA. I became a member at just three years old and learned to lift weights as soon as I was old enough to pick up a dumbbell. Becoming a trainer was just a natural progression. I was born to be a gym rat.

I don't subscribe to the notion that you have to be a gym member to get healthy. Quite the opposite: You have to figure out what you *enjoy* in order to get fit. You're not going to like the same activity as everyone else, so don't listen to all the noise when it comes to getting fit.

However, you do need to challenge your body in new and effective ways to get results. Are you a goal-oriented person? Do you feel best in the mornings or evenings? What activity would you like to try? What inspires you when it comes to getting up and moving? Perhaps it's swimming, cycling, entering a race, taking a yoga class, or trying something adventurous like trapeze (this is on my to-do list for the very near future). Sometimes, I even go to the playground that's not too far from my condo and climb the monkey bars. Or swing. Or go down a slide. It brings me back to those elementary school days when all I had to worry about was completing my homework and finishing the contents of my brown bag lunch.

Throughout my life, I've been a gymnast, a sprinter, a weightlifter, a dancer, and a boxer. I became a certified group exercise instructor and a personal trainer. I delved into nutrition, took every seminar imaginable, and became a certified nutrition specialist in plant-based nutrition, sports nutrition, and fitness nutrition. All the while, I exercised six days per week. Over the years, I've found exercises my body responds to. For now, they feel good, but as Alex and I enter the next phase of our lives, I'm sure we will start thinking more about maintaining our fitness levels instead of working out intensely—such is the nature of physical activity as we age.

When I got pregnant, my "tough" exercise principles were challenged, but I didn't stop the habit of movement that I loved. I eased up on the intensity but still managed to go to the gym six days per week, up until labor. Every morning, my husband would hit snooze on his alarm clock, screaming that his eyes were broken. We would lie there, entwined with our twin, floral Boppies (yes, he insisted on us buying *him* a body pillow after he tried mine).

Still in a half-haze of sleep, we would feel around for our puppy, to make sure she hadn't suffocated during the night. And then, with effort, I would heave myself up to a sitting position, feeling the weight of my still-sleeping daughter shift inside of me.

With the quiet familiarity of our set routine, we would slip into workout clothes, eat our hefty bananas, and head to the car. Some people marveled that I had the discipline to get up at 6:00 a.m.—no matter what—and go to the gym. But, for me, it was the one time of the day I got to spend, uninterrupted, with my husband.

On the drive, we would talk about our weird dreams the night before, our little aches and pains, our plans for the day, what workouts we were going to do, and what to eat for dinner.

Once at the gym, I was tortured. Tortured because I was limited in my movements—something as foreign to me as learning I was pregnant. (I love exercise like people love cake.) I dreamed about burpees and pull-ups, about having a good sweat and the endorphin rush that comes with it. It always motivated me in a way nothing else could.

Instead, during my pregnancy, I backed off the intensity. I strength trained three days per week and did cardio the other days. But every morning I entered that gym, I felt jealous: jealous of my husband moving his fit body, jealous of all the others lifting weights and sweating profusely. Still, with a hand on my belly, I reminded myself of what was truly important—my daughter's health—and I stuck with it. And because I stayed active and strong, I believe it helped me focus on my goals during my 52-hour labor and during my post-delivery. I eased back into going to the gym two weeks later and have since returned to my challenging workouts.

As my story shows, exercise doesn't have to be a dreaded addition to a busy schedule. It can be a natural part of life, no matter how many children you have, how exhausted you are, or how demanding your job. After all, even if you've never exercised a day in your life in the traditional sense, you must move to get through your day. And once you are able to find something you love, it's amazing what a natural part of your life it can (and should) become. Perhaps you traipse to and from the city all day, taking stairs, walking to lunch meetings, etc. This is exercise. Perhaps you are a stay-at-home mom and are on your feet all day, bending, scooping, lifting, and cleaning. This is exercise. Perhaps you go for a run every morning before the day's demands, regardless of weather or circumstance. This is exercise.

Exercise should be just as important as your job or eating healthy. It's an insurance policy against disease and a decreased metabolism. We are made to move and to move often. This doesn't mean going to the gym every day if that's not feasible or what you like to do. Cleaning, walking, yoga, dancing, biking, taking the stairs, yard work, and even caring for a child are activity enough. Getting fit doesn't have to be complicated. Simply take the guesswork out of it and find what you like and what works for your lifestyle.

However, you might have a gym membership and want to use it. Are you someone who, every time you step into the gym, looks around aimlessly and wonders what to do? Should you hop on a treadmill, sit on a machine, or reach for the dumbbells? What if you want to take a class but are too intimidated? What if you don't even want to go to the gym, and want to use your body weight for a workout? What is the absolute best workout you can do? If these are your questions, then search no further. In this chapter, I'll show you unique workouts that will have you covered on every level, no matter your fitness goal.

While there are numerous ways to work out, there's definitely a key to unlocking your best body—it's about experimentation. As with eating, there's no one right way to exercise. While someone's physique may respond beautifully to yoga or dance, another's might prefer boxing techniques or strength training.

With the workout principles in this chapter and the arsenal of exercises on pages 255–281, you can explore which movements really feel good and make a difference for your body. You can achieve a top level of fitness by using your own body weight, modifying the tough exercises, or even progressing to an advanced level. It's all about finding the type of exercise that works well with your body.

SELF-ASSESSMENT: YOUR WORKOUT NEEDS

Before you read the rest of this chapter, ask yourself the following questions.

1. *Do I go to the gym? Do I like the gym? If I go to the gym, do I do the same things over and over again?*

2. *Do I get bored easily?*

3. *Am I a beginner? Can I not afford a gym, or do I feel intimidated in a gym?*

4. *Am I a morning person or a night person?*

EVALUATE YOUR ANSWERS

If you go to the gym and tend to do the same routine over and over again, try a class. Go swimming. Try an adventure race or triathlon. If you need to be held accountable, have a friend train with you, or send out a mass email to see about getting a group together. If races aren't your thing, try a yoga class, a personal trainer, an adult gymnastics class, a dance class, or a type of martial arts.

If you are a beginner or feel intimidated at a gym, start with an exercise video in your living room or use the exercise arsenal on pages 255–281 to throw together a challenging workout in your own home, since most of the exercises can be performed with your own body weight. Figure out something you'd like to do, and then research online the best videos for that activity. If you know you won't stick to a video, go for walks. Set a timer to get up every hour and do something—walk to a co-worker's desk, walk a flight of stairs, complete a chore, do some squats and push-ups, etc. Or hire a trainer to come to your home. Just make sure you are moving for at least an hour every single day.

Wherever you work out, figuring out when you have the most energy is key to sticking with an exercise program. If you promise yourself you're going to wake up every single morning and exercise five days per week, but it's impossible for you not to hit snooze on the alarm, then be realistic. Exercise when you feel the strongest. This is different for everyone. You're more apt to stick with a program if you follow your body's natural rhythm.

General rule for activity: There are infinite ways to be active, and you don't have to devote your life to a gym to become fit. If you hate weights, don't lift weights. If you aren't motivated by running, don't run. If you want to try yoga but aren't flexible, ease into it with some planks and gentle stretches. If you don't have time for a 45-minute workout, opt for an intense 10-minute session instead.

Power Vegan Workouts

I am going to take you through my top workout techniques, which have worked for myself, athletes, overweight individuals, beginners, and thousands of clients over the years. Each individual exercise is explained in more detail in the appendix of this book. You can try one or all of them. Stick with a workout program for four to six weeks until you reach a plateau or want to change it up. In this way, you have countless options when it comes to your workout.

WORKOUT TIPS

Remember, there are no rules, but try to heed the following as you perform the workouts in this chapter:

> **Pay attention to your form.** I cannot stress this enough. Form is crucial to completing any exercise routine properly. You can do 100 squats, but if you're doing them improperly, without the right muscles engaged, then you're wasting your time and risking injury. If you're unsure of any exercise, pay attention to the photos and explanations in the Appendix (see pages 255-281), check out videos online, and don't be afraid to ask someone for help.

> **Engage your core.** What is your core? It's your entire midsection (including your lower back, pelvic floor, and hips), and should be an active part of whatever exercise you are doing. By "engaging" these muscles, or locking them into place, you protect your lower back and set the stage for a more functional exercise.

> **Breathe.** Exhale on the hardest part of the exercise (or exertion) and inhale on the easier part. If you're doing a push-up, for example, exhale when you're pushing up to the starting position and inhale on the way down. Breathing is imperative for supplying oxygen to your muscles and keeping your heart rate under control. I always tell clients as they increase their intensity to try to keep their breathing steady. Find spots within the exercise to recover. Breathing properly makes a world of difference and can shoot your fitness through the roof.

In addition to following the tips above, modify your workouts with these suggestions, tailored to individual levels:

If you're a beginner: Cut the reps in half, scale back the weight, and pay special attention to form. Don't attempt some of the more advanced movements until you're comfortable with the technique of any given exercise. You can always modify an exercise to suit your needs.

If you're intermediate: Challenge yourself by mixing up your routines and trying new movements or workout patterns. By the end of your workout, your muscles should be fatigued.

If you're advanced: If you want to rev up these workouts even more, utilize the patterns and reps in unique ways. For instance, on workouts that have a rep pattern of 12–10–8–6, 21–15–9, or 10 down, once you finish the last set, work your way back to the top. So, if you do 12–10–8–6–8–10–12, you can play with the weights and challenge your body even more. Or throw several different workout programs together in the same workout. It's all about muscle confusion to garner results.

Fighter Circuit

Even if you're not a fighter or have no interest in becoming a fighter, you can still incorporate tried-and-true movements that will whittle your core, enhance flexibility and speed, and make your body leaner and more efficient.

FIGHTER EXERCISES TO CHOOSE FROM

Bear Crawl (page 256)

Drop Squat (page 262)

Full Bosu Sit-Up (page 263)

Get-Up (page 264)

Hip Escape (page 267)

Knees (page 268)

Medicine Ball Sprawl (page 270)

Punch (page 272)

Resisted Knees (page 272)

Resisted Knees with Sprawl (page 273)

Shoulder Throw (page 275)

Thumbs Up (page 280)

SAMPLE FIGHTER CIRCUIT

Pick 5 of the exercises listed previously. Perform each exercise for 1 minute, then rest 1 minute after the entire circuit is complete. Repeat entire circuit for 45 seconds, rest for 45 seconds, and then repeat the entire circuit for 30 seconds per exercise.

CrossFit

CrossFit is the principal strength and conditioning program for many police academies and tactical operations teams. It incorporates different repetitions, body weight exercises, weight-bearing exercises, and tailored workouts to get you into peak condition in a short amount of time. For this section, I'm scaling back the weight and instead focusing on anaerobic activities that people can complete with just their bodies or a few pieces of equipment.

CROSSFIT EXERCISES TO CHOOSE FROM

Box Jump (page 257)   Mountain Climber (page 270)

Burpee (page 259)   Pull-Up (page 271)

Man-Maker (page 269)

SAMPLE CROSSFIT CIRCUIT

Perform the above exercises for 21 reps, then 15 reps, then 9 reps.

Power

Powerlifting has gotten a bad rap over the years (mainly due to grunting men who lift massive weights, guzzle gallons of water, and walk around the gym unable to put their arms by their sides due to the size of their overgrown muscles). In this workout, we are taking the best and most functional "power" movements, and letting you gradually progress to a weight that is comfortable. Women should not be afraid of weight. It takes *years* of heavy weight training (and sometimes supplements) to develop "bulky" muscles. Often, women actually don't lift *enough* weight to challenge their muscles or promote lean muscle definition. Incorporating strength training can alter your physique in numerous positive ways. Always ease in, check your form, and then gradually add weight that is challenging but not impossible. You should not feel any strain when you perform these movements.

POWER EXERCISES TO CHOOSE FROM

Clean and Press (page 261)

Clean and Press from Knees (page 261)

Deadlift (page 261)

Deadlift from Knees (page 262)

Hang Clean (page 266)

Hang Clean from Knees (page 266)

Hang Clean into Reverse Lunge (page 266)

SAMPLE POWER CIRCUIT

Pick 3 or 4 exercises, such as Hang Clean, Clean and Press, and Deadlift. Perform 6–8 reps of each exercise. Perform 3–4 sets of each exercise grouping.

Tabata

Tabata is a well-known technique in the fighting community, where entire workouts can be created around this 4-minute principle of work. Tabata works as follows: 4 minutes of activity comprised of 20 seconds of high intensity and 10 seconds of rest repeated 8 times through. You can perform Tabata with anything: sprints on a treadmill, squats, push-ups, rows, burpees, planks, and even in spin class. It is a principle you can throw into your routine whenever you want to mix it up. It comes especially in handy when traveling or when you have no equipment at all.

TABATA EXERCISES TO CHOOSE FROM

All (pages 255–281)

SAMPLE TABATA CIRCUIT

Choose 5–10 exercises and perform Tabata with each of them.

Core Training

A strong, healthy core is imperative for a strong, healthy body. The core can be involved in everyday exercises, from sitting, standing, lifting, and bending to yoga and sports. For this section, I am highlighting my favorite core exercises, which intensely work the midsection and will reap the most benefits in the least amount of time.

CORE EXERCISES TO CHOOSE FROM

Bear Crawl (page 256)

Burpee (page 259)

Cable Twist (page 260)

Full Bosu Sit-Up (page 263)

Full Partner Twisting Crunch (page 263)

Get-Up (page 264)

Hip Escape (page 267)

Inchworm (page 268)

Knees (page 268)

Mountain Climber (page 270)

Plank Jack (page 270)

Plank Mogul (page 270)

Plate Drag (page 271)

Spider Plank (page 278)

Twisting Reverse Crunch (page 281)

SAMPLE CORE CIRCUIT

Pick 3 exercises. Perform each for 90 seconds, then 60 seconds, then 30 seconds. Or pick 2 exercises and perform each for 2½ minutes.

1,000-Rep Workout

1,000 reps is a lot. Yes, this is true. For many, there will never be a need to do 1,000 reps of any exercise—ever. However, if you want to get through a workout and "blast" your body in a new and different way, the 1,000-rep workout will achieve this immediately. You can choose 10 different exercises, and then perform 100 reps of each before moving on. If 100 reps in a row is too much, perform 25 reps before moving on to the next exercise, and then go back and complete the entire circuit 4 times through. Pick exercises you know you can modify or progress as time goes on and you get stronger. You can do a full-body workout with this circuit or break it into body parts for an upper-body or lower-body blitz.

1,000 REP WORKOUT EXERCISES TO CHOOSE FROM

All except powerlifting movements

SAMPLE 1,000 REP CIRCUIT

Pick 10 exercises. Perform each exercise for 100 reps (try to get 100 reps in 2½ minutes) and then move on. If this is too much, perform 25 reps of each exercise before moving to the next, and repeat circuit 4 times.

Boot Camp

Boot camps often conjure people in the military being yelled at by drill sergeants. While this is traditionally where boot camp workouts are used, the principles they instill are for everyone: functional movements using body weight and high-intensity interval training. By incorporating short, intense bursts of activity with short recovery periods, you can increase endurance, power, and strength and get your workouts done in less time. I am including my favorite boot camp movements for a functional, intense workout that can last 10 minutes or an hour—depending on what you have time for that day.

BOOT CAMP EXERCISES TO CHOOSE FROM

Burpee (page 259)

Chest Tap Push-Up (page 260)

Handstand Push-Up (page 265)

Kamikaze Push-Up (page 268)

Knees (page 268)

Lateral Shuffle (page 269)

Man-Maker (page 269)

Mountain Climber (page 270)

Plate Push (page 271)

Prisoner Jump Squat (page 271)

Prisoner Squat (page 271)

Pull-Up (page 271)

Punch (page 272)

Renegade Row (page 272)

Smith Machine Pull-Up (page 278)

Slap Push-Up (page 278)

Towel Row (page 280)

SAMPLE BOOT CAMP CIRCUIT

Pick 10 exercises. Perform each exercise in a row for 2 minutes, then 90 seconds, then 1 minute.

Rep/Tempo

Oftentimes, all your workout needs is a bit of alternation, namely in the rep or tempo category. If you've been doing 3 sets of 10 reps for as long as you can remember, it's time to make a change.

- 21–15–9: Pick a group of exercises. Perform each exercise for 21 repetitions, then 15 repetitions, then 9.
- 7 reps for 7 rounds: Pick a group of exercises. Perform each exercise for 7 repetitions. Complete for 7 rounds.
- 5 reps for 5 rounds: Pick a group of exercises. Perform each exercise for 5 repetitions. Repeat for 5 rounds.
- 12–10–8–6 reps: Pick a group of exercises. Perform each exercise for 12 repetitions, then 10, 8, and finally 6 repetitions.
- 8–6–4 reps with a 6-second hold between each set: Pick a group of exercises. Perform each exercise for 8 reps and, on the last repetition, hold the hardest part of the exercise for 6 seconds. Repeat the exercises for 6 repetitions, then hold for 6 seconds on the last rep. Finally, repeat the exercises for 4 repetitions, holding on the last rep for 6 seconds.

REP/TEMPO EXERCISES TO CHOOSE FROM

All (pages 255–281)

SAMPLE REP/TEMPO WORKOUT

Perform the following 4 exercises for 5 reps for 5 rounds:

Kamikaze Push-Up (page 268)

Mountain Climber (page 270)

Drop Squat (page 262)

Decline Spider Plank (page 262)

Perform the following 3 exercises for 7 reps for 7 rounds:

Single-Arm Barbell Chest Press (page 276)

Hip Escape (page 267)

Broad Jump to Walk-Out Push-Up with Bear Crawl Back
(page 258)

Perform the following 3 exercises for 12 reps, then 10, 8, and 6:

45-pound Plate Push (12 pushes on each leg) (page 271)

25-pound Plate Drag (page 271)

Pull-Up to Burpee (page 271)

Body Part Split

Many people prefer to separate their body parts, working them
on specific days. However, this can get boring. I am including
some new and creative ways to keep muscles constantly confused
(which is essential for building strength) and to fatigue the body
in a short amount of time. You can include different reps and use
any of the programs discussed previously. Whatever body part split
you choose, pick a few exercises from the Arsenal of Power Vegan
Exercises and challenge yourself by using different reps or workout
principles to achieve your desired goal.

SAMPLE BODY PART SPLIT EXERCISES TO CHOOSE FROM

All (pages 255–281)

SAMPLE BODY PART SPLIT WORKOUT FOR SHOULDERS/ HAMSTRINGS

Perform 12 reps, then 10, 8, and 6 of the following 3 exercises:

Clean and Press (page 261)

Deadlift from Knees (page 262)

Hang Clean into Reverse Lunge (page 266)

Perform 5 reps for 5 rounds:

Punch (page 272)

Bear Crawl forward and back (page 256)

Scarecrow (page 273)

Perform each exercise for 12 reps, then 10, 8, and 6:

Squat with One-Arm Twisting Row (page 279)

Figure 8 (page 263)

Single-Leg Deadlift (page 277)

10 Down

One of the most effective workouts around, 10 down utilizes a high-rep principle with any exercise to get the most out of a workout when you are limited on space (perfect for hotel rooms). You perform 10 reps of an exercise, then 9, then 8—all the way down to 1. You can do this with virtually any of the routines or exercises in this chapter. Focus on what your specific goals are and what you want to achieve.

SAMPLE 10 DOWN EXERCISES TO CHOOSE FROM

All (pages 255–281)

SAMPLE 10 DOWN WORKOUT

Perform 10 reps of all of the following exercises in a row, then go back and repeat for 9, 8, 7, 6, 5, 4, 3, 2, and 1:

Prisoner Squat (page 271)   Mountain Climber (page 270)

Prisoner Jump Squat (page 271)   Burpee (page 259)

Slap Push-Up (page 278)   Plank Jack (page 270)

No matter which of these workouts you choose, the point is to have a plan when you exercise. We don't go into the grocery store to be completely blindsided, with no clue of what we want or need to buy (or maybe we do—and that's part of the problem). It's the same for exercise. We often want to get healthier or stronger, but we don't know *how*. We don't understand the structure of our bodies or how we might react (or not react) to certain activities. So we hire a trainer or take a class and entrust others with our health.

Take your health into your own hands, because no one knows what your body needs as well as you. While I think certain trainers are incredibly motivational, and can even be lifesavers, there comes a point when you have enough tools in your arsenal to create activities that suit your lifestyle. Before launching into any of these Power Vegan exercises, examine what you are currently doing and find ways to ramp it up.

My top tips for improving your training?

- **Change the reps.** If you typically perform 3 sets of 10–15 reps, try any of the following rep changes with any grouping of exercises (as previously explained in the rep/tempo workout principles on page 150):
    - 7 reps for 7 rounds (Pick several different exercises. Perform 7 repetitions of each exercise in a row. Repeat for 7 rounds.)
    - 10 reps for 10 rounds (Pick several different exercises. Perform 10 repetitions of each exercise in a row. Repeat for 10 rounds.)
    - 21–15–9 reps (Pick several different exercises. Perform 21 reps of each exercise, then 15 reps, then 9.)
    - 5 reps for 5 rounds (Pick several different exercises. Perform 5 repetitions of each exercise. Repeat for 5 rounds.)
    - Tabata: 4 minutes (20-second interval followed by 10-second rest. Repeat 8 times to equal 4 minutes.)

    You can use your own body weight, resistance bands, weights, or stick to plyometrics, which are fast and powerful movements, such as Jump Squats, Box Jumps, Jumping Lunges, etc. You can take Squats, Push-Ups, Pull-Ups, Step-Ups, or Jump Squats and make a tough workout with any of the aforementioned rep variations.

- **Get off the machines.** Machines aren't intrinsically bad, but they're not going to let you follow a natural movement pattern, as you do in life. Think functional activity. Is rowing 300 pounds really the best way to get a strong back, or should you attempt to do a pull-up instead—an activity that can aid in a host of other activities in daily life? Think about why you do the exercises you do. Are they serving you in daily life and your everyday activity?

- **Do interval training.** If you're one of those people who stays at the same intensity during workouts, it's time to shake things up. If you're doing cardio, ramp up the intensity for 30 seconds, back off for a minute, and then repeat this sequence for the duration of your workout. The same goes for lifting. If you are a regular weightlifter, throw in 5 repetitions of Burpees, Pull-Ups, and Box Jumps for an added dose of intensity. Get those fast-twitch muscle fibers firing. When we train,

we sometimes limit ourselves to specific movements. Break
outside your comfort zone. Just make sure you are executing
exercises safely. Know your limitations.

■ **Eat proper pre- and post-workout fuel.** Eat simple sugars
before and simple sugars with a bit of protein directly after, and
then a more stable meal an hour after that (see Chapter 8). If you
do a protein shake after you workouts, cut the protein in half,
throw in a piece of fruit, and see how you feel. Pay attention.

■ **Try something new.** Often, ramping up your fitness means
trying something different. Opt for an activity you've always
wanted to try: dancing, Pilates, boxing, cycling . . . the list is
endless. See what feels good to your body and then try that for
a specific amount of time.

Bottom Line

Remember that our bodies adapt and need consistent change to reach
the proper gains. Don't be afraid to challenge yourself in new and
exciting ways.

QUICKEST WAY TO INCREASE ENDURANCE: TRY TABATA.

CHAPTER 11

Eat to Cure Your Ailments

"Part of the secret of success in life is to eat what you like and let the food fight it out inside."

—MARK TWAIN

In our society, it's common to go to the doctor when you experience a physical ailment. More often than not, the symptoms are addressed and you are given a prescription. After you peruse the list of unfortunate side effects (that can sometimes take up an entire page), you might experience some of them yourself, which can be worse than the initial problem you went in for. You might even go back to the doctor and get a *new* pill. And thus the cycle continues, until you don't know what it feels like to just be healthy without the constant aid of medication (or the innate fear of getting sick).

Bottom line? Pills don't solve medical issues. They can *contain* issues, but they don't cure them. We've become so far removed from our bodies—from tuning in, from providing proper nutrition, rest, and happiness—that we forget we can cure almost anything with what we eat. Yes, food is *that* powerful. And so are our bodies, if we just give them a chance to heal.

Fact: According to a Senate investigation discussed in *Diet for a New America* by John Robbins, medical doctors receive less than *three* hours of nutrition training in medical school.[28] While many doctors are knowledgeable in terms of what your body needs, many are not well versed in nutrition.

So, the question remains: Why do we live in a society where we let professionals who often have less knowledge than us about our bodies tell us what to eat, how to live, how to move, and what to be concerned about?

While doctors are mandatory in so many situations, oftentimes, when you are experiencing common, everyday ailments, you'd be surprised at how easily you can fix them on your own. It's time to take responsibility for your health and physique and learn to put all of your new habits together in a sensible way that equals one thing: *success.*

One easy way to do this: Instead of popping pills, open your refrigerator. While everyone has complaints when it comes to their physical and emotional lives—"I'm exhausted," "I need to lose five pounds," "I feel bloated"—the answer isn't always in the medicine cabinet. Simple, powerful foods can make you feel amazing. They can erase exhaustion, extra weight, bloating, and other symptoms. It's just about choosing the right foods for you.

But how do you know when you are experiencing a more serious ailment as opposed to one that can be fixed by food? Pay attention. A little experimentation goes a long way. If your food or lifestyle changes aren't working, however, it's always good to seek medical attention to check for an underlying condition.

Top Ten Ailments and How to Fix Them

The following are ten common ailments and how to fix them with food. Want to go the extra mile? Peruse the exercise and lifestyle info, as well as the common foods to avoid. For the exercises, aim for three sets of 10 to 12 repetitions, or study Chapter 10 and incorporate the movements into your everyday workouts.

While everyone is different, when you combine healthy diet, exercise, and lifestyle components, you will be amazed at what balance you can achieve.

I HAVE LOVE HANDLES

People joke about love handles and muffin tops, but excess fat, especially around your waist, can lead to a host of diseases and issues if not careful. While you can't "spot reduce" when it comes to weight loss, there are certain foods and exercises that can target a soft middle. Using your entire core when you move; eating enough of the "good" fats, such as those in avocados, nuts, seeds, coconut, hemp, chia, and flax; cutting down on processed, fatty foods; and ingesting plenty of fibrous, watery fruits and vegetables can get rid of love handles once and for all.

> *Eat:* Raw, unsalted, soaked nuts; seeds; quinoa; millet; buckwheat; cucumbers; berries; asparagus
>
> *Sweat:* Plank Jack, Hip Escape, Burpee (see Appendix)
>
> *Live:* Drink plenty of water to flush toxins from the body. Reduce stress by laughing and spending time with loved ones. Lighten up. Find humor and happiness in everyday situations, as stress can raise cortisol levels, which often translates to belly fat. Depression can also lead to unwanted weight gain and lethargy. Reduce heavy restaurant dining (skip the bread basket and heavy extras, such as butter and creamy salad dressings).
>
> *Avoid:* Excess dairy, alcohol, processed meats, oils, butter

I FEEL SLUGGISH

Feeling sluggish on the outside often has to do with what's going on *inside* your body. If you are constantly feeding your body processed foods, heavy meats, dairy, excess sugars, and caffeine, you can experience a sluggishness that is hard to shake. If you're not eliminating at least three times per day or not getting enough quality grains, fiber, and healthy fats, you can feel lethargic. Sweating, while not scientifically proven to release toxins, is still key to that endorphin rush and that glow that make you feel wonderful.

> *Eat:* Vegetables, fruits, quinoa, millet, buckwheat, teff, seeds, nuts, beans

Sweat: Step-Up into Reverse Lunge, Handstand Push-Up, Plate Push (see Appendix)

Live: One of the first signs of being tired is dehydration. Drink plenty of water, especially when you first wake up. Try to down a glass of water before every meal.

Sweat. Literally. If you don't sweat easily when exercising, layer your clothing to raise your body temperature. Make sure you are working out at a challenging level and not coasting through your workouts. Use your entire body instead of isolating body parts. Opt to work out in the morning if you can, to stimulate blood flow and keep your metabolism stoked all day. If you don't have time to work out, take the stairs or walk. Make movement part of your daily routine.

Always eat breakfast and afternoon snacks, which can help you avoid that midmorning or afternoon slump. Think about fueling your body all day to give you energy, so you don't have to rely on sugary snacks and caffeine.

Avoid: Excess caffeine, alcohol, cookies, crackers, pasta, gluten (if you have a sensitivity)

I FEEL IRRITABLE

Bad moods or negative attitudes can strike at any time. One minute you can be on a high, the next you could kill someone. What you eat has a direct connection to how you feel. Sugar and caffeine can give you bursts of energy and then make you plummet (Exhibit A: children eating sugar). Eating foods that induce sustainable energy is key; so is doing quick bursts of exercise to boost mood. Eating too many refined foods and indulging in sugar and alcohol (which is a depressant) can cause bad moods as well. Aim for mood-enhancing nuts, B vitamins, grains, and fibrous vegetables to boost serotonin, which is a mood regulator.

Eat: Fruits, vegetables, walnuts, dark chocolate, cocoa or cacao, nutritional yeast, coconut oil

Sweat: Bridge, Sprint, Punch (see Appendix)

Live: Laugh. Talk. Figure out what is making you irritable. Is it food related? Work related? Relationship related? Do you constantly complain and discuss what you don't want to happen? Or do you try to surround yourself with positive people? Do you keep everything inside and let it explode, or do you rationally discuss your issues? Do you have too much on your plate? Focus on pinpointing and remedying the issues at hand.

Avoid: Alcohol, caffeine, sugar

I HAVE NO SEX DRIVE

Sex drive can be affected by a host of issues: what you eat, how much you exercise, your partner, and hormonal fluctuations throughout the month. However, by tweaking your diet, aiming for intense bursts of exercise, and making time for pleasure, you can keep your sex drive constant all month long. Any foods or exercises that increase blood flow will stimulate your sexual organs, leading to that desire to get between the sheets.

Eat: Watermelon, chocolate, asparagus, pumpkin seeds, bananas, garlic, avocado, maca

Sweat: Spider Plank, Man-Maker, Bear Crawl (see Appendix)

Live: While sex is amazing, sometimes it can be the last thing on the to-do list. See Revive Your Sex Drive, on the next page, for tips on how to make it a priority.

For one week, try to connect every day. This can be through foreplay, intimacy, or just paying attention to each other's needs. Have a conversation about it. Ask how you might improve your physical relationship so it can lead to a better emotional relationship. Even if that's completely different terms for each of you, you can find a way to meet in the middle.

Avoid: Alcohol, candy, fatty meats, cheese, soy, sugar, and too much technology, especially before bed

REVIVE YOUR SEX DRIVE

Use these quick tips to get back in the mood:

■ **Be intimate with your partner.** Though men and women are different and some men will probably tell you they prefer sex over intimacy, intimacy goes a long way to get anyone in the mood for sex. What does intimacy mean for you and your partner? Ask each other. Is it holding hands? Rubbing your partner's back before bed? Smothering each other in kisses? Taking a walk? Turning off the television and actually talking? Examine your current relationship and see where more intimacy might fit in. A simple touch, kiss, or even a kind word can sometimes be just as satisfying as rolling in the sheets. (Yes, really.)

■ **Have lots of foreplay.** Many couples I talk to have one complaint: There's no foreplay. He wants to jump straight to sex. She won't go anywhere below the belt. Women don't often "turn on" as easily as men, and men don't always want to go straight to work. The solution? Don't be subtle about what you like. In fact, taking your partner's hands (or face) and showing them exactly what you mean will be thrilling beyond belief. But, that goes both ways. Do you expect your partner to do all the work? If there's something that drives them crazy (in a good way), do it without asking. Tease your partner. Be aggressive. Make them beg for you. It's surprising what a turn-on that can be.

■ **Have morning sex.** There's something about being intimate before the day has completely started—before workouts, deadlines, traffic, or kids—that is golden. Even if you're still half asleep and you have morning breath, simply back up against your partner and let your bodies do the rest. There are no distractions or excuses. It starts the day off right every time.

■ **Be selfless.** If you think your partner is unsatisfied, do a favor and don't have them "reciprocate." Not only will this be a surprise, it might turn you on as well. Wanting to please our partners should be just as important as getting pleased. We are sexual beings, yet somehow sex gets pushed to the back burner as we sit in front of the television or spend countless hours on Twitter or Facebook. Take 20 minutes to connect with your partner instead.

I HAVE BAD SKIN

Hormones, stress, too many processed foods, and harsh chemicals can all cause bad skin. The more antioxidants you consume (think fruits and vegetables), the more vitamins and minerals will make their way to your complexion, improving its radiance. Reducing stress and outside toxins can help target bad skin (if you can't eat it, don't put it on your skin). Reducing highly processed, fatty foods can also help as well, as can exfoliating dead skin cells regularly. In addition, always drink plenty of water.

Eat: Berries, vegetables, quinoa, oats, walnuts, almonds, cashews, pumpkin seeds, berries, kiwis, zucchini, bananas

Sweat: Bronco Burpee, Inchworm, Broad Jump (see Appendix)

Live: Exfoliate. Removing dead skin cells allows skin to breathe. Instead of using harsh chemicals or trying to pick one of the endless products out there, make your own exfoliant combining sugar, lemon or lime juice, and a bit of oats and honey. Mix together and gently scrub your face.

Experiment with other items in your kitchen to get the softest, most radiant skin possible. Look at all the products you put on your face. Read every ingredient. Nix anything with numbers, dyes, or fragrances—these are all irritants and should be avoided.

Look at your shampoo and conditioner, makeup, and facial cleansers. Do they have fragrance in them? Can you pronounce half of the words? If not, consider switching to more natural products or even making your own. Coconut oil makes a perfect body moisturizer and hair conditioner.

Have you washed your pillowcase lately? If you are a side sleeper, oils from your hair and hair products can build up on the pillowcase and cause breakouts. While sweating is wonderful for skin, make sure to always shower immediately after a workout. If you drink alcohol, try to down a glass of water before every drink, as alcohol depletes the skin (and wreaks havoc on the liver).

Avoid: Oils, butter, cheese, candy, sodas, caffeine, alcohol

I HAVE BRITTLE NAILS/DRY HAIR

Your skin, nails, and hair can tell you a lot about your health. If your nails continually break, you may not be getting enough micronutrients and calcium from plants (which is absorbed much more easily than calcium from animal sources). The same goes for your hair. If your diet consists of coffee and fast food, or you often go hours between meals, you could be ruining your insides—and your outward appearance will show it.

> *Eat:* Collard greens, spinach, strawberries, figs, white beans, fortified nondairy milk, nuts, seeds, sea vegetables

> *Sweat:* Shoulder Stand, Handstand, Reverse Crunch (see Appendix)

> *Live:* Look at the ingredients in your shampoo and conditioner. Most shampoos and conditioners on the market contain detergents, surfactants, alcohol, artificial fragrances, preservatives, and silicon.[29] Scroll through the ingredients and avoid words you can't pronounce, numbers, or capital letters like PEG. Instead, opt for a short ingredients list with natural oils, berries, or juices. All ingredients should be recognizable and from natural sources. Do you wash your hair every day? If so, reduce to a few times per week to prevent breakage and dry hair. Do you wear your hair up every day? This can cause severe breakage. Once a week, make your own deep conditioner with olive or coconut oil. Rinse your hair with beer, which will give it a beautiful shine. Opt for a shower filter to remove unwanted toxins and chlorine from the water you bathe in, which can help your skin, hair, and nails. If you constantly wear nail polish, try to cut back, as this can cause the nails to become brittle and break.

> *Avoid:* Chemicals, smoke, processed foods, caffeine, sugar

I HAVE NAGGING ACHES AND PAINS

Aches and pains can come from a variety of sources, including weakened muscles surrounding a joint, overuse, improper activity throughout the years, or too many inflammatory foods. Many aches and pains can be virtually erased with the right diet and by focusing on strengthening the surrounding muscles. In addition, fixing your Omega-3 to Omega-6 ratio can virtually eliminate inflammation in the body. Vitamin C has been known to reduce wear and tear on joints, which keeps free radicals from ravaging the body and helps in the production of collagen, a known protector of cartilage and bones.

> *Eat:* Hemp, flax, nutritional yeast, seeds, nuts, beans, kelp, ginger, garlic, berries
>
> *Sweat:* Single-Leg Deadlift, Scarecrow, Incline Push-Up (see Appendix)
>
> *Live:* Pay attention to how you feel after you eat, especially when eating gluten and sugar. If you indulge in a sugary treat and wake up the next day with aching joints, you may need to cut back on the sugar. The same goes for bread. Make sure you are getting enough Omega-3s, which are natural inflammation fighters.
>
> Are you fueling properly after workouts? Are you working on flexibility? Do you schedule rest days after your workouts, or do you not give your body time to recover? Perhaps investing in a foam roller to break up scar tissue induced by workouts can help your nagging aches and pains. Do you wear comfortable shoes or are you always in high heels? Are you well hydrated, or do you live on coffee and tea? Look at your everyday lifestyle to try to pinpoint what could be hindering you from feeling good.
>
> *Avoid:* Cooking oils, sugar, trans fats, dairy, meat, alcohol, gluten, refined grains

I HAVE ALLERGIES

Food allergies and other types of allergies can strike at any time. While some food allergies are unfixable, some can actually be completely eliminated by shifting what you eat and therefore getting rid of reactions such as congestion, sneezing, and rashes. Cutting back on refined grains, dairy, wheat, soy, nuts, and sugar and incorporating more whole foods can often help you pinpoint and reverse allergies. Sinuses can become clear. Often what you assume is a cold is really just an aversion to certain foods.

Eat: Vegetables, fruits, pseudograins, seeds

Sweat: Towel Row, Renegade Row, Thumbs Up (see Appendix)

Live: Think about getting an air filter in your home to target airborne toxins, which can bother sinuses. Dust often. Invest in a good vacuum that doesn't stir up too much dirt and dust. Remove pet dander. Eliminate heavily processed grains and sugars that can often trigger allergies, and opt for dairy-free options to see if you feel better. Focus on eliminating one element at a time so you can figure out what might be making you feel bad.

Avoid: Dairy, wheat, gluten, nuts, soy

I FEEL BLOATED

Bloating can be caused by carbonated drinks, too much fiber, sugar-free gum, drinking through straws, hormone fluctuations, or a possible food intolerance, such as dairy or gluten. When it's "that time of the month," cutting back on processed foods and excess caffeine, while drinking a lot of water and eating water-packed fruits and veggies, can help reduce bloat for women. However, bloating can also be a symptom of more serious internal inflammation. Look at your diet closely when you bloat to see if you can pinpoint the culprit(s).

Eat: Zucchini, kale, asparagus, grapefruit, pumpkin seeds, water

Sweat: Knees, Plank Mogul, Cable Twist (see Appendix)

Live: Start paying attention to how you feel after you eat. Are you bloated? Energized? Exhausted? Every time you have ice cream, do you get a stomachache or have bathroom issues? Often, you can figure out what your body does and doesn't like just by paying attention. Listen to every signal to avoid uncomfortable digestion. When are you most bloated? Is there a trigger? If you eat out a lot, always remember to ask the restaurant to go light on the salt. Drink water and eat bloat-reducing foods.

Avoid: Gluten, dairy, meat, caffeine, soda, gum, alcohol, sodium

I FEEL STRESSED/EXHAUSTED

Stress is literally a killer. When we are stressed at home, at our jobs, or in our relationships, we can become overwhelmed and chronically tired. We don't often get enough "primary food" in terms of happiness, fulfilling careers, and a balanced home life. We often reach for the quick fix when it comes to food, which can contribute to exhaustion and stress. Not making enough time for yourself, not eating right, or not exercising can also cause stress.

Make sure you are eating energy-inducing foods. While caffeine might seem like a good idea, it is actually stealing energy your body doesn't have. And you will crash every time. Opting for grains like quinoa, which is loaded with iron, B vitamins, and protein, can keep you energized and help keep stress at bay. Eating walnuts, which are full of mood-enhancing omegas, and even throwing some dark chocolate or vegan chocolate into your buckwheat pancakes, can help boost mood and ease stress.

Eat: Fruits, vegetables, green juices, walnuts, quinoa, nutritional yeast, oats

Sweat: Reverse Burpee, Downward-Facing Dog, Lateral Hop (see Appendix)

Live: When do you find yourself stressed or tired? Do you wake up exhausted? Perhaps your sleep is to blame. Americans are notorious for not getting quality sleep. According to research first brought to my attention in a seminar by Brendan Brazier, if you can remember your dreams, you're not hitting the good delta sleep we all need. Most bodily repairs happen while sleeping, so getting good sleep quality (over quantity) is key. For quality sleep, reduce light from the television, computer, and phone before bed. Play relaxing music or take a bath. Get in a nighttime ritual to reduce stress.

When do you find yourself stressed at work? If you can, try to delegate the tasks that bog you down to someone else so you can focus on top priorities. Check your email once every hour instead of constantly (which can reduce stress and that sense of urgency). Focus on one task at a time instead of five at once.

At home, figure out what the "triggers" are that make you crazy. Is it that the house never stays clean? That your partner won't help? Rather than getting angry, realize that there is a solution to every problem. Calmly approach the issue and enlist the help of others. Don't feel like you have to do it all yourself, or that someone else won't do it right (yes, that means you, control freak). Realize that if someone completes something in a different way than you doesn't make it wrong—it's simply their process.

Try to be a non-interferer with your children, your partner, and at your job and see how stress and exhaustion might lessen. If you do find yourself at a breaking point, practice deep breathing. Take five minutes to check out, listen to your favorite song, or go for a quick walk. Try to laugh.

If exhaustion is your problem, make time to exercise. Though this might sound backwards, boosting blood flow and getting an endorphin rush can supply energy, not rob it. Ease in with simple movements and increase from there.

Avoid: Caffeine, sugar, processed foods

Bottom Line

Whatever your ailment or issue, take the time to examine your habits and make changes through diet, exercise, and factors in your environment. Notice the "avoid" lists in this chapter. See any similarities among the lists? Try backing off some of the common culprits and see if one issue or several disappear. As always, if you are suffering from a severe issue and lifestyle changes don't work, it is always a safe bet to seek professional help.

QUICKEST WAY TO BOOST YOUR MOOD: DRINK A GLASS OF WATER AND GO FOR A SHORT WALK.

CHAPTER 12

Overcoming Any Obstacle for a Healthy Life

"A man can live and be healthy without killing animals for food; therefore, if he eats meat, he participates in taking animal life merely for the sake of his appetite."

—LEO TOLSTOY

By now you know what to eat, how to prepare it, what to stay away from, and most importantly, why. However, this isn't a foolproof strategy to ensure success. After all, many of us know what to eat. If it were that easy, we'd all be fit and healthy. In everyday life, resolve is lost, issues come up, finances falter, fatigue sets in, and we inevitably revert back to what we know best: routine.

For example, how do you maintain a proper eating balance when schedules get in the way, when you don't have groceries on hand, when you lose your willpower, when you have nagging injuries, or when you are just tired of thinking about it?

Look no further than this simple fix guide. With real solutions, you can pave the path for success before you ever embark down the road of dietary manslaughter. (Yes, this is a real thing. I have lived and learned.)

Top 12 Common Excuses and How to Fix Them

Here are the 12 most common reasons for not maintaining a healthy lifestyle. Find your own issues in the following list, and read on for easy ways to overcome them.

I HATE HEALTHY FOOD

First, define what healthy food means to *you*. If you were forced to eat Brussels sprouts and cabbage as a child, then you might have an aversion to these foods. Luckily, there's a plethora of healthy foods to choose from, and regardless of what popular food brands, the dairy industry, or the meat industry want you to believe, healthy food usually doesn't come from a package. It comes from the ground.

Think about the foods you enjoy. If you have a sweet tooth, there's a good chance you'll like fruit. If you like smoothies, chances are you can hide a fistful of spinach or kale in there without even tasting it. Do you like pasta? Opt for quinoa, brown rice, mung bean, or buckwheat soba noodles. Can you handle a salad? Load it with tomatoes, avocado, celery, broccoli, and pumpkin seeds. If you like burgers and fries, make small, progressive changes. Perhaps a bison or turkey burger and sweet potato fries are the initial transition before switching to a delicious black bean burger and side salad. Take baby steps so it doesn't feel like deprivation. Search for quick, easy recipes for foods you love with the freshest ingredients.

Think about the small ways you can incorporate healthy foods into your diet. Expand your knowledge of what's healthy and what's not (your body definitely knows the difference). Find vegetables, fruits, grains, seeds, and nuts that you actually like. This might take a bit of experimentation, but do what works for you. Don't like fresh fruit? Opt for dried, but look for natural, organic dried fruits that have no extra sugar added. Don't like nuts without salt? Make your own trail mix and add high-quality sea salt to the mix. It's all about shifting your mindset and being open to change.

Most important? Think *simple* in terms of healthy food. It doesn't have to be complicated or on some top-ten list to be healthy. If you load up a salad with bacon, cheese, croutons, egg, and a heavy dressing, what's the point? Swap with avocado and seeds and then make a creamy dressing with tahini and a fresh herb like dill. Fresh and simple go a long way for optimal health.

It's also important to look at the foods you don't like and figure out how they were prepared. Instead of simply saying "I don't like that," perhaps try it prepared a different way. For instance, if you hate zucchini, try using it in place of pasta noodles and cover it with an enjoyable, healthy tomato sauce (see page 219). If you don't like apples, perhaps sprinkle them with cinnamon and bake them, or have them fresh with a nut butter. It's about giving healthy foods another chance in a different way to see if your tastes may have evolved over the years.

Oftentimes, if you cut back on salty, greasy fare and introduce healthier foods, you will find that your taste buds completely change and acclimate to the taste of fresh foods, without all the unnecessary extras like salt, butter, and heavy oils getting in the way.

I DON'T KNOW HOW TO COOK

It's common to eat out these days, order in, or just grab prepackaged meals because you are exhausted, you don't have time, or you can't fathom the thought of making dinner *on top* of everything else you have to do. If you don't know how to cook or you just don't want to cook, fear not: There are plenty of ways you can get the nutrition you need—and not from the freezer section.

If you absolutely refuse to even boil water or spend 10 minutes in the kitchen, a little detective work will be required. You need to read labels on all prepackaged items you buy. Look for natural ingredients with words you can pronounce. Shorter lists are always better.

The best bet is to purchase items that don't have an ingredient list at all, or only have one ingredient. Try to stick with organic whenever possible. If you're eating out, ask to go light on the oil and salt, and always ask how your food is prepared. Even if the menu claims it's healthy, it's usually not. Most chefs have some sort of legume or grain on hand. Ask for a side of beans and rice with a salad and you have a perfect little meal, packed with antioxidants, fiber, and protein. When ordering an entrée, ask to double the veggies and skip the often-buttered bread or unhealthy appetizers. When you order in, don't forget to ask for your items steamed, baked, and made with no salt (you can always add your own at home). Get dressings on the side.

If you are willing to do a little work in the kitchen without using serious knife skills, opt for easy meals. If you like salads but hate to chop, purchase pre-chopped produce (just know you will pay a little more). Buy easy grains and beans that can be made in short amounts of time (boiling water is all it takes). Invest in a slow cooker and load it up with beans, grains, and veggies before you leave the house. You'll come home to a simple, delectable meal.

Peruse recipes that have five ingredients or less. Make easy granola (see page 220) or no-bake energy bars (see page 233). And most importantly, figure out what you hate about cooking. Is it that you can't chop, or you despise the long list of ingredients? You can make virtually any healthy meal with just a few staple ingredients. If you have them on hand, you can throw together meals in no time. And while your food is cooking, clean up so you won't have a pile of dishes staring back at you.

Also think about the culprits that tend to lead to your demise: What do you crave at night? What do you love to eat? When do you lose your resolve? Try to cover all your bases so the excuse of "I don't cook" doesn't derail your healthy plans. And, if you just won't ever be open to cooking, aim for mostly raw foods. Eat raw at home and cooked foods when you're out. Eating easy salads, smoothies, raw energy bars, cold soups, wraps, sandwiches, fruit, and soaked nuts and seeds not only helps you avoid cooking, but boosts nutrition as well.

I CAN'T CONTROL MY CRAVINGS

Cravings and American fare go hand in hand. You can't turn on the television or drive 10 miles without seeing signs for fast food. We've come to "crave" foods because it's what we've been introduced to—not what our bodies really want.

First, you have to figure out what you are craving. Sweet? Salty? Savory? Something in between? Going back to Power Vegan rule three: Figure out what you love and learn to make it healthier. If you crave ice cream, opt for an almond milk or coconut milk variety. Or even make your own using dates and cocoa or cacao powder (see recipe on page 230). Like cookies? Make a healthier version. Love pizza? Opt for a cheeseless variety and load it up with veggies and nutritional yeast or a soy-free, dairy-free cheese like Daiya (if you have soy allergies). You don't have to give up your cravings—just alter them. It's not sustainable to say "I'm giving up sugar forever" (trust me, I've tried), so find ways to indulge your cravings where guilt and feeling bad aren't involved. What can you feel good about eating?

Second, when does your craving hit? Is it when you're sitting in front of the television, bored, or when you are genuinely hungry? Did you skip lunch and now you've got donuts on the brain? Are you really, truly hungry, or are there other feelings involved? (For example, do you feel like you deserve something sweet/salty/savory as a reward?)

The trick is to find something that is truly satisfying and isn't junk food. Once you get a handle on what you crave, when you crave it, and how much it takes to satisfy the craving, you can get your food desires under control. As Joshua Rosenthal states in *Integrative Nutrition*, "[a] sugar craving is simply the body asking for energy."[30] Ask yourself what fuel your body really needs right now. Sometimes, people think they are hungry when they are really just thirsty. So down a full glass of water. Craving something in the afternoon? Perhaps you did not get enough sustenance at lunch. (I will not suggest chewing gum as a substitute for snacking, as there are more chemicals in gum than you can imagine. Read the ingredients and then throw it away.) Bored? Go for a quick walk.

What are the consequences for your body if you eat sugar every night? Though you may not pay now, you will always pay later. Think about the integrity of your food and why you even crave the foods that you do. How much of it is learned behavior?

Figure out what your health is worth to you and go from there. How many cookies have you had in your lifetime? Is it *really* worth it to have one more? How are you going to feel 20 minutes after you eat it? Guilty? Mad? If you feel good about your decision, eat it. If not, don't avoid your cravings, but try to take steps to curtailing them.

Craving still there? Here are some rules:

> **Try to give in to cravings just once or twice per week.** If you eat ice cream every day, chances are you're not going to feel great. Pick two days, such as Wednesdays and Saturdays, where you can indulge in something you really want. Then plan activities around your craving, so you don't just eat and go to sleep.

Try to indulge during the morning or the middle of the day, versus at night, when you are most sedentary. If you indulge during the earlier part of the day, you have a better chance of using the food as fuel. If you are the type of person who feels guilty after the fact, then go for a walk or engage in some sort of activity (sex, anyone?).

Try to satisfy your craving with the smallest amount. If you're craving something sweet, try a piece of fruit or just one square of dark chocolate and then make yourself a cup of decaffeinated hot tea. Sipping on something warm can sometimes do the trick. And while fruit is a great option, it's still loaded with simple sugars, which usually fuels your body for activity. If you're just going to be sedentary, these health foods will be stored as fat (much like any food you eat that isn't burned). If fruit or chocolate doesn't do it, then indulge in what you want, but try to have half the amount. Share it with someone else. Eat slowly. Drink plenty of water, then focus on a task that doesn't involve food.

Tame your sweet/salty/crunchy cravings the easy way. In addition to trying the delicious sweet recipes in this book (see page 220), try the following:

- Frozen grapes
- Frozen nondairy yogurt topped with sliced berries and walnuts
- Vegan hot cocoa (mix cocoa and water or nondairy milk and add a bit of honey or agave if necessary)
- Dark chocolate
- Vegan desserts (while these shouldn't be a daily staple, they will definitely do the trick—more and more bakeries and restaurants are serving vegan alternatives, so if you want a big slice of cake, you can have it)
- One cup (110 g) granola (see page 220) or store-bought cereal topped with unsalted almonds, berries, and nondairy milk (read all ingredient labels on store-bought cereals, watching out for empty-calorie products, sodium, and sugar)
- Homemade trail mix with granola, nuts, dried fruit, and vegan or dark chocolate

- Pita chips with homemade hummus (you can make your own pita chips by purchasing fresh pita, cutting into triangles, and baking so there's no added salt or oils)
- Organic kettle popcorn or bagged varieties

If you have a more specific craving, see below.

- If you're craving cereal, try: Almond and Sunflower Seed Granola (see page 220). While no store-bought cereals are very healthy, some brands are better than others. Don't have 20 minutes to make a batch of granola? Check out the less processed brands in the grocery store. Look for high-fiber content (at least four grams), lower sugar, and just a few ingredients. Top with fresh berries and some hemp or almond milk for a decent nighttime snack.
- If you're craving chocolate, try: Dark Chocolate, Chia, and Cherry Pecan Bar (see page 232). A square of dark chocolate usually takes the edge off, but if just one won't do, make a decadent dark chocolate bar or even throw together a chocolate panini with two fresh pieces of bread, a basil leaf, and dark chocolate. Heat on a griddle and enjoy!
- If you're craving ice cream, try: frozen nondairy yogurt. Pop your favorite flavor of nondairy yogurt into the freezer. Mix in some cocoa or cacao powder. Top with fresh fruit and enjoy a creamy, frozen treat that will quell your craving for ice cream. Or opt to make your own nondairy version at home (see page 230).
- If you're craving pasta, try: zucchini pasta or brown rice pasta. Zucchini pasta mimics the taste of pasta for a fraction of the calories and carbs. Toss with some olive oil, pumpkin seeds, and tomatoes and you have a nice healthy treat. If you want something more substantial, go for the brown rice pasta (or other pasta options listed on page 101).

I EAT TOO MUCH

This is an easy fix. Eating too much of the wrong foods is one thing, but eating an abundant amount of the right foods is another. Unhealthy, processed, heavy foods are dense but not nutritionally beneficial. They fill up the stomach but are less satisfying, allowing you to stuff more and more in until you feel terrible.

When you eat fiber-rich, nutrient-dense foods, you are satisfied quicker, but can eat more often. You don't have to count calories or track your fat intake. Much like an infant, you eat when you're hungry and stop when you're full. You learn to tune in to your body and let go of all the set rules we've been taught about when to eat, how to eat, and most importantly, what to eat.

If you start filling up with fibrous, natural foods, you will notice you can eat more while feeling amazing and energetic. The moment you stop thinking in terms of calories and start thinking in terms of eating nutrient-dense food, you can eat more and get full faster. But remember: It's easy to eat six handfuls of nuts per day or an endless amount of pita chips just because you think they're healthy. Pair empty-calorie foods like chips with a bean dip or hummus. With nuts, try to eat a water-packed piece of fruit and find your "satiation" point.

Don't mindlessly eat—be aware of what you're eating and why. If you're going to sit on the couch for the entire night, do you need a giant serving of nuts as a post-dinner snack? Or a nondairy milkshake? Probably not. Fuel your activity. If you want the milkshake, have it and then go for a walk. Or have a glass of hot tea and then assess what you want and why. Start paying attention to what your body really wants, and more importantly, what it needs.

Also look at what you eat the most of, and when. Is it pizza? Is it when you've had a few cocktails? When you're eating out? When you've skipped lunch? Pinpoint the triggers and then try to keep yourself from eating mindlessly. Remember that purchasing bags of cookies or chips sets you up for failure. These are completely empty calories, and it's often impossible to just eat one. If you really love chips, make your own pita chips, or even take it a step further and opt for sweet potato chips or kale chips. If you love cookies, make a big batch of your own (10-minute commitment, tops—see page 225). That way, when you reach for something you're craving, you can ingest better ingredients, which means a happier, healthier you.

If you tend to eat the most when you've skipped meals, try to pack snacks to prevent the binge. If you scarf food down with friends or while standing up, be mindful. Put your fork down between every bite, drink water, and chew. Focus on each bite and enjoy the food you're eating—

you will almost always stop short of full if you pay attention to what you're eating.

I'M NOT HUNGRY

If you're not hungry, you have probably slowed your metabolism. Do you skimp on breakfast? Do you only eat two or three times per day? Our bodies are made to burn fuel, but they have to ingest fuel to burn it. Are you perpetually busy? Do you glance at the clock and realize five hours have passed and you haven't had water or food? You can slow your metabolism to a crawl if you consistently skimp on meals.

Look at your lifestyle. If you don't have time to eat breakfast, have a "to-go" item ready and waiting. Try one of the quick breakfast recipes in Chapter 13. Smoothies take less than a minute to make. Bake muffins the night before or have a quick muesli that you can eat cold in the car. Pack fruit, nuts, seeds, salads, homemade energy bars—foods that you can eat on the go. Stash these in your office, your car, your purse, or at the gym. Never have an excuse to not eat. The more you eat, the more you will burn (but no, this doesn't mean gorge yourself seven times per day).

Set a reminder on your phone or computer every 3.5 hours that it's time to eat. Even if that meal is some dried apricots and almonds, it's better than eating nothing.

Often, when people start eating more often, their energy soars, they don't need caffeine, and they shed unwanted weight. All by doing one thing: eating regularly. Try to get on a schedule with your eating. Your body will thank you.

I DON'T HAVE ANY FOOD IN THE HOUSE

Welcome to most of America, where we get home at the end of the day and ask that dreaded question: "What's for dinner?" You rummage through cabinets and wonder how on Earth you don't have anything to eat, when you just spent a fortune at the grocery store. How can you not have any food in the house? Having a plan of action for these times is a good idea. If you do, chances are you can pull together a pantry meal or something quick without having to break the bank on takeout.

Do you have beans on hand? Lettuce? Grains? A healthy pasta? You can make a quick meal in 15 minutes or less if you purchase these staple ingredients and always have them in your kitchen. If you really want to do takeout, see what you have around the house that can make it healthier. Ordering Chinese? Cook up some quinoa or brown rice, lightly water-sauté some veggies, and throw both in your dishes when your takeout food arrives.

Making a menu on Sundays and then shopping for the week can also solve this problem. If you can plan your breakfasts, snacks, and dinners for three to four days, you will be ahead of the game. Think about big pots of soup or chili that you can make in bulk and have for leftovers the next day (or freeze and have for weeks or months at a time). Think about simple, four- or five-ingredient meals. If you make a soup one night, you can add a healthy grain or pasta the next to create a slightly "elevated" meal for no money and minimal effort.

You can also set up an automated grocery delivery service, or join your local community-supported agriculture (CSA) program, both of which will deliver groceries to your door every week so that you don't have to even think about it. If you really are out of fresh food, making easy pantry meals from beans, rice, and canned tomatoes also works in a pinch. Always have healthy takeout menus ready to go, so you have options if the refrigerator is empty.

I DON'T HAVE TIME

Time—that elusive concept that seems to escape us all. We fill our days so tightly that we rarely have time to do the things we want to do. We spend eight hours per day at our jobs and countless hours on chores and errands, and yet limit time with loved ones to those rare moments or special vacations. Often, we are "too busy" to get coffee with a friend or break free from our routine, pack a picnic, or even relax under the sun.

Every day, we have choices about what we want and how we plan to get it. In terms of health, you are the only one who can make time for those choices. Health should be a top priority, not something that's pushed to the back burner.

Exhaustion plagues most Americans. We stack so many things on our plate, we have to schedule sleep and sex. There's very little spontaneity to the way we live anymore. From morning to nightfall, we work, move, text, email, drive, and talk our way to exhaustion. We sit and sit and sit and tell our bodies that they are sedentary, when in fact they are dying for movement. The first line of defense if you're tired? Move. Even a quick walk will get the blood flowing. Second: Drink a glass of cold water (and even splash some on your face, which will get adrenaline pumping). Third: Figure out when you have the most energy, and attack your eating plan for the day. Plan what you want to eat, and make it happen—whether that's having your groceries delivered, enlisting the help of a loved one, or even looking up healthy restaurants in your area.

Then look at what you *do* have time for. Can you boil water? Then you can make a big pot of healthy grains and beans. Do you have 10 extra minutes at night to prep for the next day? Make a large salad and divide up your snacks for the next day. Do you have time to make a grocery list? Personalize your list and print off numerous copies so you can just check off the items you need. Look at what you can do and how you want to eat. Do you eat a lot of takeout? If you're watching one of your favorite shows at night, can you get up during the commercial break and pack some healthy snacks and a lunch for the next day? Can you peruse easy, five-ingredient dinners and walk to a grocery store during your lunch hour? Can you enlist the help of others in your household? If you can't prep food or go to the store on Sunday, hit the store on a weeknight after dinner. Don't think you have to do it all, or that it has to be complicated. If you have to choose between making a quick, healthy 10-minute meal or doing another load of laundry, make the meal. Chores will always be there—but you can literally shift the way you feel in an instant with what you put into your body.

Are you a planner? If you can pinpoint the issues that prevent you from eating healthy, you can put a plan in place to eradicate those issues.

Now ask yourself: What do I *not* have time for? If it's grocery shopping, get your food delivered. Many services offer recipes on their sites and will keep a tab on what you usually order so there's minimal time involved in getting your groceries. If it's prep work you don't have time for, purchase sprouted grains or lentils that only take five minutes to boil, or pre-made salads and chopped veggies. Buy all-natural dips to throw together with some kale chips or veggie slices. Get ingredients for smoothies. Look for organic energy bars with the most natural ingredients possible.

FOOD GOES BAD NO MATTER WHAT I DO

We've all been there. You stock up on fresh produce with the best intentions, only to find a soggy plastic bag in the refrigerator a week later, full of what used to be something healthy. The average American wastes hundreds of dollars a year on discarded, unused food—usually produce. Families discard about 470 pounds of food per year. Nationally, we dump about $43 billion worth of food per year![31] Since produce isn't cheap, it's best to arm yourself with the following hard and fast rules when purchasing it, so you don't run into this problem.

See what ingredients you use the most. Do you consistently buy apples, bananas, lettuce, etc.? Figure out how much you go through per week and ration out your produce so you have just enough. Look at your pantry staples (the ones that you actually use) and purchase items in bulk so you don't have to always run back to the store. What about the items that have been sitting there forever? Were they impulse purchases? Did you have a recipe in mind that didn't work? If they're past their expiration dates, toss them. If they're not, try to use them up before purchasing a slew of new items that might go bad.

Have a specific recipe in mind. Don't shop blindly. You might pick up those berries or that zucchini thinking you're going to use them, but chances are, if you don't have a meal in mind, they'll go to waste. Go to the store with a prepared shopping list and only buy enough for the recipes you'll make, and a few other items you know you will use. It's easy to go for those "two-for-one" deals, but don't do it unless you know how you can use those items.

Only purchase enough for a couple of days. If produce perpetually goes to waste in your household, only buy enough food for a couple of days. Purchase items for breakfast, lunch, dinner, a few snacks, and that's it. While you may have to pop into the store a bit more, you can ensure that items won't rot.

Chop and store produce the moment you get home. Prep salads, chop veggies and put them in new bags, store apples on a separate shelf so as not to spoil other produce from the release of their ethylene gases (ripening agents that cause rapid decay of certain fruits and vegetables)—the minute you get back. It's easy to purchase items and then pop them in the fridge and forget about them. Instead, as soon as you get home, wash, rinse, and chop the produce so it's ready to use.

Keep produce at eye level. It's easy to forget about fruits and vegetables if they're at the very bottom of the refrigerator in plastic bags. As soon as you get home, clean and store in proper produce bags (or skip the bag altogether) at eye level, either on the countertop or in the refrigerator. This way, you'll know what you have and how much.

Survey the refrigerator every few days. See what you might be able to blend into a smoothie, freeze, or add to your meals. Keep an eye on the items you may have forgotten about. Every time you're packing a snack or throwing together a meal, search your produce to see what you might add. Or better yet, make a big batch of veggie soup or tomato sauce and store in the freezer, so you will have something delicious on hand when you're tempted to order takeout. Just be aware of what you bought and when you might be able to use it.

Store produce properly. Beat the odds and know how to store your produce to make the most of its shelf life. Sometimes this is as simple as knowing which items to refrigerate, which to leave out, and which never to put in the same drawer together (due to that tricky ethylene gas).

Following this handy guide, you can extend the shelf life of your fresh produce.[32]

REFRIGERATE

Apples

Apricots

Cantaloupe

Figs

Honeydew

DON'T REFRIGERATE

Avocados

Bananas

Nectarines (unripe)

Peaches

Pears

Plums

Tomatoes

KEEP THESE AWAY FROM OTHER ITEMS

Apples

Bananas

Broccoli

Brussels sprouts

Cabbage

Carrots

Cauliflower

Cucumbers

Eggplant

Lettuce and other leafy greens

Parsley

Peas

Peppers

Squash

Sweet potatoes

Watermelon

If you know you're not going to take the time to separate produce, invest in produce bags or other products that extend shelf life.

The key is to know what to eat first based on how quickly it spoils, and what you can leave a bit longer. Thanks to *Vegetarian Times* and the research of Marita Cantwell, PhD, a postharvest specialist at the University of California, Davis, here's an entire week of what to eat (assuming you went shopping on Sunday):[33]

EAT FIRST:

SUNDAY TO TUESDAY

Artichokes

Asparagus

Avocados

Bananas

Basil

Broccoli

Cherries

Corn

Dill

Green beans

Mushrooms

Mustard greens

Strawberries

EAT NEXT:

WEDNESDAY TO FRIDAY

Arugula

Cucumbers

Eggplant

Grapes

Lettuce

Limes

Mesclun

Pineapples

Zucchini

EAT LAST:

WEEKEND

Apricots

Bell peppers

Blueberries

Brussels sprouts

Cauliflower

Grapefruit

Leeks

Lemons

Mint

Oranges

Oregano

Parsley

Peaches

Pears

Plums

Spinach

Tomatoes

Watermelon

AND BEYOND

Apples (remember to keep them separate)

Beets

Cabbage

Carrots

Celery

Garlic

Onions

Potatoes

Winter squash

I DON'T HAVE THE MONEY

Eating power foods doesn't have to break the bank. Yes, healthy, organic food *is* often more expensive, but it's an insurance policy for your health. (Pay now or pay later.) Still, there are ways to save.

Search for coupons for boxed or packaged items. Always purchase produce that's in season (see Chapter 2). Frequent your farmers' market to get what's local. Not only will the taste blow you away, you can get more for your money and ingest fresher food that hasn't been shipped as far.

Rather than purchasing ingredients for a complicated recipe, purchase just a few items for several meals so produce doesn't rot in the fridge. You could get beans, rice, and some veggies for a Mexican bean bowl. Throw the leftovers over greens the next day for a Mexican salad. Make a quick soup for dinner by using a veggie broth and a few vegetables.

You can have enough fresh food to last the whole week for a very reasonable price—just know what to buy, when to buy it, and where you can cut back. For instance, instead of purchasing expensive nut butters, simply make your own by grinding nuts in a food processor. Instead of buying nondairy milk, blend nuts and water and strain through a nut bag or sieve.

If you are on a strict budget, adhere to the following shopping principles:

Buy from bulk bins. Get all of your seeds, nuts, and grains from the big bins to save you endless amounts of time and money. Invest in a big shopping trip for your beans, grains, nuts, and seeds and store for weeks or months at a time.

Research to find the cheapest organic produce. Chances are, there are markets or even services online that offer cheaper organic produce than some stores. Look into co-ops or local services that deliver organic produce straight to your door. Not only may prices be lower, but you can do all of your shopping with a click of a button—often for half of the price of fancier grocery stores. Many also offer no sales tax and free shipping. Also, those fruits and vegetables with thicker peels, such as bananas, avocados, grapefruits, and oranges, can sometimes be bought in conventional varieties without compromising your health.

Make big dinners. Making a big stir-fry or pot of soup will ensure one thing: leftovers. When you make dinner, see how the dish could be altered the next day for lunch. Could it be thrown over a salad? Made into a sandwich? Paired with some beans and quinoa? Be frugal and creative at the same time.

Plan your meals. Often we spend so much extra money on groceries and let perfectly good produce go to waste because we don't know what we're going to make before we go the store. If you can take 15 minutes on the weekend to plan your meals for the week, you can save a ton of money and avoid countless impulsive trips to the store. Make a customized grocery list (use the list of staple foods to have on hand on page 244 as a sample) and then stick to it. If you can just print off your list and keep it handy, you won't be wandering the aisles and stocking up on things you don't need.

Make a budget. Really look at where the majority of your money for food is going. Is it on eating out? Produce? Meat? Dairy? Processed foods? Keep your grocery and restaurant receipts for a month and then go over them (this can be quite shocking, so be prepared). Where can you afford to cut back or make simple changes? For instance, if you love energy bars but hate the cost, make your own. The same goes for ice cream, juices, and chips. It's so much cheaper and simpler to make giant (and healthier) batches of foods on your own than to buy overpriced options.

I DON'T HAVE ENOUGH WILLPOWER

Willpower is a finicky thing. They say it takes 21 days to make something a habit, but how do you get to 21 days, when by day 3 all you want to do is stuff your face with brownies? I can speak to this particular issue better than anyone, as I have never mastered it when it comes to sweets. I can work out six days per week. I can make myself write for hours every day. I can take care of my daughter all day every day. But after dinner, I *cannot* seem to refrain from eating something sweet.

Perhaps it's simply habit, but if so, it's one that has never been completely broken. Fruit usually fits the bill, or homemade vegan brownies or cookies. I can go weeks without sweets, but that inevitable desire rears its ugly head. And so I've realized I can *enjoy* baking something for my family. I enjoy the sensation of eating a dessert after dinner and not feeling guilty or bad the next day. I've simply changed what I'm eating so I am indulging without the "guilt" often associated with a pint of ice cream. This is how I have maintained willpower—not through deprivation, but through finding ways to adjust how I indulge.

With many of my clients, I tell them the same thing. Think about the food(s) you love more than anything. How many times have you had them in your life? What good have they brought you? *Really*? What has that pizza done for you? The ice cream? The fried food? The cheese? Why do you even love those foods? Chances are, you love the foods because you're used to them or you associate them with good times and fond memories.

The good news? You can love something healthy much more than your beloved unhealthy fare. When you eat healthy, you don't have to have "willpower." You have an abundant, limitless array of foods to choose from—sweet, salty, savory—it's all there. No matter what you're craving, there's a healthy alternative.

Make a list of the foods you can't live without—the ones you dream about, crave, and love. Then sit down with the recipes in this book and see if they cover those cravings. If not, Google quick recipes for the foods you love—chances are you can find a vegan counterpart or a meal with simpler, better ingredients that will blow your mind with its exceptional taste.

Don't want to cook? Thoroughly browse the store and read all the ingredients on the packages for the things you love. Think simple. Think minimal. And then get ready to alter your taste buds in favor of something exponentially better for you and your health.

Next, figure out when your willpower is lacking. Is it at night? During the day? First thing in the morning? After you've had a few drinks? When you're with friends? Is it a routine, like clockwork? It's Friday night—you don't want to cook, so you order takeout? And that starts the weekend free-for-all? If any of these scenarios sound familiar, experiment in the following ways:

- If you must have dessert, switch to a healthier version (see the recipes in Chapter 13 for ideas).

- If you like to eat sweets at night, try to eat something sweet after lunch to see if you're just as satisfied. Eating a dessert earlier in the day will give you more time to digest and burn it off. If this works, then try to limit the frequency with which you "need" this treat, or schedule it for after a tough workout, when your body wants to devour simple sugars.

- If you absolutely have to have something decadent, engage in physical activity after. Go for a walk. Clean. Have sex. Hit the gym. Just be active.

- If you crave takeout or a giant pizza, try to tailor your order. If you love pizza, skip the cheese or ask for a light amount of cheese, load it with veggies, and pair it with a side salad. Does that do the trick? If you want greasy Chinese, ask to go light on the salt, get the sauce on the side, and instead of the nutritionally-devoid white rice, quickly boil some brown rice or quinoa at home to pair with your dish.

- If you consistently lose your willpower when you're tired, try to rest instead. Or drink a big glass of water and see if you still want what you want. Distract yourself. Call someone on the phone. Eat a piece of fruit. Make a cup of hot tea. Don't be so quick to jump to food.

- If you lose your willpower when you're stressed, eating something indulgent isn't going to tackle the stress. Focus on what's happening with your body: raised cortisol levels and that fight-or-flight instinct. If you add a nutritionally devoid meal, you are going to make that stress so much worse, adding nutritional stress to physical and emotional stress. Try to eat something for energy, something that will calm you down. See if that does the trick.

Whatever your issue with willpower, there is a way to break it. You control every single thing that passes your lips. Ask yourself before you indulge: Is this worth it? How will I feel 10 minutes from now? Tomorrow? How many times have I had this food in my life? Is it really worth it?

If so, indulge. If not, kick the habit and try something new. Willpower is completely up to you.

I DON'T SEE RESULTS

In the United States, we expect quick fixes for our health problems, regardless of how long it took us to become unhealthy in the first place. If we don't see results, we think we're not doing things right—period.

If you work out at the gym two hours per day but eat unhealthy food, you're not going to see results. If you eat "well" but aren't active, chances are you're not going to see the types of changes your body is really capable of. Perhaps you eat well and exercise but are overly stressed. Your body will react accordingly. So, first, you have to find the trigger that is not getting you the results. Is it diet, exercise, lifestyle, or all three?

Take one area at a time and see what adjustments you can make. For instance, if you've really gotten a handle on your eating but just don't have time for the gym, carve out 10 minutes to perform simple one-minute exercises such as Squats, Push-Ups, Lunges, Mountain Climbers, and Burpees (see Appendix). Take a walk after dinner. Climb the stairs. Stretch. Stand up from your desk at regular intervals. You can easily stay active all day long with short bursts of activity. You don't have to be a gym member to be considered active.

The same goes for eating. If you kill it in the gym or are even moderately active, but you just can't get the eating right, examine what you *can* do. Can you eat two healthy snacks, a good breakfast, and a sensible lunch? If so, then ease up on yourself at dinner.

If you feel like your eating and fitness are on par, but you are stressed beyond belief or miserable in your relationship, you can release stress hormones that will wreak havoc on your body. Examine your personal life—Are you happy? Are you sleeping? Are you overworked?—and make changes accordingly. Being happy goes a long way to being healthy—it's not all about diet and exercise.

Regardless of the culprit, see where you can do better and work through your issues slowly so you can ensure lasting success.

IF I WORK OUT A TON, I CAN EAT WHATEVER I WANT

This age-old excuse is the furthest thing from the truth. The reality is we grossly exaggerate how much we actually burn while we exercise. If you moderately exercise for an hour or two, you can easily replace those calories in one meal or heavy snack. Hitting the treadmill for an hour and then eating like you just ran a marathon won't do your stomach any favors.

Eat for energy. Eat for fuel. Eat for vitality. Eat proper pre- and post-workout foods and then be sensible for the rest of the day. Sedentary at night? Taper off of sugary or complex-carb-heavy meals at dinner. Do you work out, forget to eat, and then find yourself starved? Start making it a habit to pack post-workout food to immediately fuel your body.

Start looking at the portions of the food you eat. If you like to eat a lot, make breakfast and lunch your biggest meals of the day and try to eat a smaller meal at night. Or, eat an earlier dinner and then eat a smaller snack a few hours before bed. Don't ever deprive yourself—simply look at what your body requires for exercise, plan your meals around it, and then try to see what's lacking for the rest of the day. You don't have to eat a traditional American dinner of protein, carbs, and fat—that's simply what we've been taught. See what your body needs that it hasn't gotten. Have you gotten all your vitamins and minerals? Healthy fats? Good grains? Plenty of protein? Use dinner to fill in the gaps. Try to remember that balance is key.

There's never an excuse to eat "whatever you want." As such an obese, sick nation, we don't have that luxury. We need to stop making excuses and start using common sense. Period. If you're eating more power-dense foods, you don't have to pay attention to complicated ratios. But if you work out for an hour and then go through the drive-through, you are sending your body mixed signals—signals that won't garner you health or increased fitness.

Bottom Line

The bottom line is that your success is entirely in your hands. You can't blame your lifestyle or habits, as there's literally a solution to every problem. You just have to take a little bit of time to see where improvements can be made, healthier foods can be incorporated, and your lifestyle can be slightly altered.

Regardless of what you decide, use this book as a tool for incorporating healthier foods and simple tactics into your daily life.

Remember to take it a day at a time and to continuously educate yourself about what your body needs. Drown out the diet noise. Do what makes you happy. And if you do this, you will achieve lasting results.

QUICKEST WAY TO FIX A HEALTH/DIET PROBLEM: FIGURE OUT WHAT IS HINDERING YOUR SUCCESS AND COME UP WITH THREE TANGIBLE SOLUTIONS.

CHAPTER 13

Power Vegan Recipes

"We live in an age where pizza gets to your home before the police."
—*JEFF MARDER*

Often, there's this idea that you either love cooking or you hate it—but hopefully, if you're like me, you're somewhere in between. Cooking does not have to be time-consuming or complicated. Your meals don't have to be expensive or laden with a list of ingredients a mile long.

As I've said before, the very best foods are those that have been unaltered—foods that are in their natural state. So, if possible, try to eat foods that are raw and pure the majority of the time. But when you do want to cook, land on easy, simple recipes that will satisfy the entire family with minimal preparation.

The recipes in this book are all family friendly. They are made with everyday ingredients that are easy to find. If you're interested in a raw lifestyle, check out the resources page, where you will find my favorite raw cookbooks and websites and more adventurous foods and recipes.

All recipes in this book are geared to bring you energy. They have no meat, fake meat, gluten, or dairy, and most recipes can be made in 20 minutes or less. I've tried to strike a balance between recipes for people who are seasoned in the kitchen and those for people who have never so much as cut up an apple.

Instead of the traditional breakfast/lunch/dinner/dessert format, you'll find recipes organized alphabetically and divided into two categories: savory and sweet. I am a believer that you can have pancakes for dinner or a kale and sweet potato hash for breakfast. Everyone's different, and our needs change daily.

Use these recipes as staples, and don't be afraid to experiment, add or subtract from the recipes, or try completely different combinations. See which foods make you feel great and energized.

Each recipe will make two to four servings, depending on how much you eat. If you're like my husband and me, you eat a lot, but we always manage to have leftovers.

You will also find three extras with each recipe: a power boost, a time saver, and a money saver. Whether you want extra energy, don't have the time, or need to save money but still want to eat as well as possible, peruse the suggestions to see which ones are applicable to you.

POWER VEGAN SHORTCUTS

For any of the recipes with beans or legumes, I suggest buying dried beans, soaking them overnight, and then slow-cooking them. However, as lovely as that sounds, not all of us have slow cookers or time to soak and cook dried beans. Therefore, I have specified canned or boxed beans for most of the recipes instead. I encourage you to substitute the same amount of dried, cooked beans wherever you want.

A good option is to search for canned brands that have BPA-free can linings (Eden Foods is my go-to staple), or search for companies, such as Fig Food Co., that sell boxed beans. Make sure to rinse your beans, and always look for low-sodium varieties. If you do opt for dried beans and find them supremely bland, use fresh herbs and spices or a high-quality sea salt to master the perfect taste.

Best Ways to Add Power to Any Recipe
- Throw fresh berries, seeds, sea vegetables, or greens in your dishes.
- Add a pseudograin, like quinoa, for added protein and fiber.
- Use coconut oil instead of olive or vegetable oil.

Best Time Savers

- Purchase pre-cut veggies.
- Double or triple the recipes and make giant batches of snacks, breakfasts, or entrées so you don't have to think about what you're going to eat the next day.
- Think raw. If you opt for smoothies or salads, you save an abundance of time and can often throw easy veggies, fruits, nuts, and seeds together for satisfying, quick snacks.

Best Money Savers

- Buy all seeds, nuts, and grains from bulk bins whenever possible.
- If you make a large dinner the night before and have leftovers, reheat with a hearty grain you already have on hand.
- Buy local. While organic produce is preferable, if it's shipped from Mexico or Peru, prices are inflated to include the cost of shipping. Pay attention to the labels and where your food comes from.
- Buy what's in season. Look for organic produce that's in season. However, if you want to buy organic but can't afford it, stick to the types of conventional fruits and vegetables with thicker peels, such as bananas, citrus, and avocado, where pesticides don't often penetrate as deeply.

POWER VEGAN TIP

While recipes are great, the best way I've found to approach meals is simplicity. Aim for raw ingredients as much as you can (think fresh produce and fresh salads). Think five ingredients or less. Make smoothies. Make green juices. Pop seeds and beans onto salads. See how you can make tasty treats just by blending a healthy raw sauce to go with it. You don't have to have a fancy recipe to be satisfied.

Savory Recipes

Black Bean Bowl

4 SERVINGS

4 cups (948 mL) water

2 cups (380 g) sprouted brown rice

2 (15-ounce [426-g]) cans or boxes low-sodium black beans, drained

Dried onion flakes, to taste

Paprika, to taste

1 cup (88 g) broccoli florets

1 zucchini, chopped

2 tomatoes, chopped

1 avocado, chopped

Handful raw almonds

Bragg's Liquid Aminos or coconut liquid aminos, to taste

1. In a saucepan, combine the water and brown rice. Bring to a boil, cover, and lower the heat to medium. Cook for 20 minutes, or until the rice is tender. Set aside.

2. In another saucepan, cook the beans, onion flakes, and paprika over medium heat until the beans are warm.

3. Place the broccoli and zucchini in a steamer. Steam for 3 to 4 minutes, until the broccoli is bright green.

4. Combine the rice, beans, and cooked veggies in a bowl. Add the tomatoes, avocado, and almonds. Season to taste with the liquid aminos. Serve immediately.

- -

POWER BOOST: *Sprinkle with nutritional yeast for an extra dose of vitamin B and protein.*

TIME SAVER: *When the rice has about 5–10 minutes cooking time left, toss in the broccoli and zucchini and replace the lid.*

MONEY SAVER: *Purchase conventional avocado and rice out of a bulk bin.*

Basil Hummus

4 SERVINGS

1 (15-ounce [426-g]) can or box low-sodium garbanzo beans, drained

¼ cup (59 mL) olive oil

1 clove garlic, chopped

2 tablespoons tahini

2 tablespoons fresh basil, chopped

1 tablespoon pine nuts

¼ teaspoon ground cayenne

Juice of one lemon

1 to 2 tablespoons water

Additional olive oil, for drizzling

¼ teaspoon paprika

1. In a food processor, process the garbanzo beans with the olive oil, garlic, tahini, basil, pine nuts, cayenne, and lemon. Add 1 or 2 tablespoons of water as necessary to achieve the desired consistency.

2. Transfer the hummus to a bowl. Drizzle with the olive oil and sprinkle with the paprika. Serve.

- -

POWER BOOST: *Add a vegetable to the mix, such as roasted squash or broccoli, before processing.*

TIME SAVER: *Purchase lemon juice instead of fresh lemons to avoid getting seeds into the mixture.*

MONEY SAVER: *Skip the tahini.*

Black Bean Quesadillas

4 SERVINGS

> **2 (15-ounce [426-g]) cans or boxes low-sodium black beans, drained and rinsed**
>
> **Paprika, to taste**
>
> **Dried oregano, to taste**
>
> **6 Roma tomatoes, chopped**
>
> **½ red onion, chopped**
>
> **2 garlic cloves, minced**
>
> **Kernels from 2 ears fresh corn**
>
> **3 limes**
>
> **3 avocados**
>
> **1 bunch cilantro, chopped**
>
> **4 sprouted grain tortillas or brown rice tortillas**
>
> **1 (8-oz [227-g]) package Daiya Mozzarella Style Shreds**

1. In a saucepan, combine the beans, paprika, and oregano. Cook over medium heat until the beans are warm, about 5 minutes.

2. Place the tomatoes, onion, garlic, and corn in a bowl and squeeze the juice of 2 of the limes into the mixture. Set aside.

3. In another bowl, smash the avocados and add the juice of the remaining lime and the cilantro. Set aside.

4. Flatten a tortilla. Scoop the bean mixture and the tomato mixture onto the tortilla, along with a handful of the Daiya Mozzarella Style Shreds. Fold the tortilla in half. Repeat this step with the remaining 3 tortillas.

5. Grease a griddle or skillet and place it over medium heat. Cook the tortillas for 3 to 4 minutes on each side, until slightly browned.

6. Top with the avocado mixture and extra tomato mixture and serve.

- -

POWER BOOST: *Add fresh shiitake mushrooms or portobellos for a meaty texture and a dose of vitamin D.*

TIME SAVER: *Scoop cold beans into the tortillas with the Daiya and the tomatoes instead of cooking the beans first.*

MONEY SAVER: *Buy fresh, organic pico de gallo instead of making the tomato mixture.*

Chickpea–Red Pepper Salad

4 SERVINGS

2 (15-ounce [426-g]) cans or boxes low-sodium chickpeas, drained and rinsed

2 red bell peppers, finely diced

1 bunch cilantro, chopped

1 bunch flat-leaf parsley, chopped

3 cloves garlic, minced

Juice of 1 or 2 lemons

1 tablespoon olive oil

1. Toss together all the ingredients in a large mixing bowl.

2. Chill the mixture in the refrigerator up to 2 hours to let the flavors meld, and enjoy!

- -

POWER BOOST: *Toss in walnuts and sprouted quinoa for a dose of Omega-3s and fiber and a huge boost of extra protein.*

TIME SAVER: *Toss the mixture together at night and divide it into containers so it will be good to go for the week's lunches.*

MONEY SAVER: *If you have coconut oil on hand, warm it to room temperature and use it in place of the olive oil, which can be quite pricey.*

Chopped Salad with Dijon Dressing

4 SERVINGS

SALAD

3 stalks celery

1 bell pepper

1 cucumber

1 head romaine lettuce or red leaf lettuce

1 large carrot

1 tomato

⅓ head of red cabbage

½ red onion

Handful cilantro

DIJON DRESSING

1 tablespoon olive oil

Dash Dijon mustard

Juice of one lemon

1. Finely chop all the salad ingredients and place them in a bowl.

2. Prepare the dressing by mixing together all the ingredients. Toss the dressing with the salad. Serve!

- -

POWER BOOST: *Add bean sprouts (or any sprouts) to the salad.*

TIME SAVER: *Don't have time to chop produce? Pop all the ingredients in a food processor and pulse 3 or 4 times.*

MONEY SAVER: *Always make your own salad dressings with oil, lemon and/or apple cider vinegar, and spices. They are cheaper and tastier, and you can make just the amount you need.*

Citrus Gazpacho

4 SERVINGS

>   **1 large grapefruit**
>   **1 cup chopped cherry tomatoes**
>   **1 avocado, peeled and chopped**
>   **½ cup (119 mL) reduced-sodium tomato juice**
>   **½ cup (75 g) chopped red bell pepper**
>   **¼ cup (59 mL) reduced-sodium vegetable broth**
>   **¼ cup (33 g) peeled and chopped cucumber**
>   **2 tablespoons chopped red onion**
>   **2 tablespoons chopped cilantro**
>   **2 tablespoons chopped fresh basil**
>   **2 cloves garlic, minced**
>   **2 tablespoons fresh lime juice**

1. Peel, section, and seed the grapefruit. Chop the sections and place them in a bowl.

2. Add all the other ingredients. Gently mix. Cover the gazpacho and chill for 4 hours before serving.

- -

POWER BOOST: *Add some fresh dandelion greens.*

TIME SAVER: *Throw all the dry ingredients into a food processor and pulse a couple of times instead of chopping.*

MONEY SAVER: *Make your own tomato juice from fresh tomatoes.*

Coconut Curry Vegetable Soup

6 SERVINGS

  6 to 8 red potatoes

  2 tomatoes

  1 or 2 yellow or orange bell peppers

  1 eggplant

  1 onion (red or yellow)

  1 stalk broccoli

  1 small cauliflower

  1 bunch bok choy

  Handful mushrooms (shiitake or portobello)

  1 head garlic (optional)

  Olive oil or coconut oil, for drizzling

  4 cups (948 mL) coconut milk

  Curry powder, to taste

  Paprika, to taste

  ½ cup (12 g) fresh basil, chopped

  Fresh cilantro for garnish (optional)

1. Preheat the oven to 350°F (180°C). Rinse and roughly chop the potatoes, tomatoes, bell peppers, eggplant, onion, broccoli, cauliflower, bok choy, and mushrooms. Peel a few cloves of the garlic and leave them whole.

2. In a bowl, toss all the vegetables after drizzling with the oil. Arrange them on a parchment-lined cookie sheet.

3. Bake until the potatoes are well done (about 30 minutes). While the vegetables are baking, cook the coconut milk with the curry powder, paprika, and fresh basil in a saucepan over medium heat.

4. Once the vegetables are done, pour them into the coconut milk and stir until the soup is heated. Serve immediately, garnished with the fresh cilantro.

- -

POWER BOOST: *Add a sea vegetable, like dulse, to the vegetable mixture.*

TIME SAVER: *Choose vegetables that don't require a lot of chopping if you are short on time.*

MONEY SAVER: *Pick only two or three vegetables to save you time and money.*

Collard Enchiladas

8 SERVINGS

ENCHILADAS

2 cups (474 mL) water

1 cup (190 g) sprouted brown rice

1 summer squash (green or yellow)

1 (15-ounce [426-g]) can or box low-sodium black or pinto beans, drained and rinsed

2 cloves garlic, minced

Dried onion flakes, to taste

Dried oregano, to taste

Paprika, to taste

1 bunch cilantro, chopped

Juice of 3 limes

1 bunch collard greens, ribs removed

SAUCE

2 tomatoes, chopped

1 (4-ounce [114-g]) can green chiles

¼ cup (59 mL) olive oil

2 tablespoons white vinegar

1. Preheat the oven to 350°F (180°C).

2. In a saucepan, combine the water and brown rice. Bring to a boil, cover, and lower the heat to medium. Cook for 20 minutes, or until the rice is tender.

3. Once the rice is done, add the cilantro and the lime juice and set aside.

4. In a skillet, sauté the squash and beans with the garlic, onion flakes, oregano, and paprika.

5. Combine all the sauce ingredients in a blender. Blend them until smooth and transfer to a saucepan. Heat the sauce for 5 minutes over medium-low heat.

CONTINUED ON NEXT PAGE

6. Lay the collard greens flat. Spoon the rice and bean mixture onto the collard greens. Roll them up like small burritos.

7. Place the enchiladas side by side in a glass baking dish and cover the dish with aluminum foil.

8. Bake the enchiladas for 30 minutes. Pour the sauce over the enchiladas halfway through the baking time. Serve hot.

- -

POWER BOOST: *Throw in some spinach or kale with the beans and squash for an added dose of greens.*

TIME SAVER: *Buy an organic chile sauce and forgo making your own.*

MONEY SAVER: *Purchase dried beans instead of canned. Soak and cook the beans the night before and pop them in the enchiladas the next day.*

Kale and Sweet Potato Hash

4 SERVINGS

> **1 teaspoon coconut oil**
>
> **½ white onion, diced**
>
> **3 garlic cloves, diced**
>
> **1 sweet potato, peeled and cubed**
>
> **1 large bunch kale, ribs and stems removed, leaves rinsed, and cut into 1-inch strips**
>
> **½ cup (80 g) grape tomatoes, halved**

1. Place a pan lightly greased with coconut oil over medium heat. Add the onion and garlic and sauté for a few minutes.

2. Add the sweet potato and kale, cover, and cook for 5 minutes. Toss in the to-matoes. Stir the mixture until the sweet potatoes have the desired texture. Serve.

- -

POWER BOOST: *Throw in some lentils or beans for an added dose of protein.*

TIME SAVER: *Instead of cutting the kale, prepare it ahead of time by ripping it from the ribs, rinsing it, and setting it aside so it's ready to go.*

MONEY SAVER: *Always opt for sweet potatoes, which are grown in the United States, as opposed to yams, which are usually shipped farther (and cost more).*

Kale and Garlic Chive Pesto Salad

4 SERVINGS

⅓ cup (48 g) almonds

3 cloves garlic, minced

1 bunch garlic chives, minced

2 tablespoons olive oil, divided

½ leek, thinly sliced

Juice of one lemon

1 bunch kale, finely chopped

1 cup (30 g) mesclun greens

Currants, for garnish

1. In a dry pan over medium heat, toast the almonds for about 5 minutes.

2. In a food processor, combine the almonds, garlic, garlic chives, and 1 tablespoon of the olive oil. Process until well combined.

3. In a sauté pan, combine the remaining tablespoon of olive oil, the leek, and two heaping spoonfuls of the almond and chive mixture. Cook over medium heat for 1 to 2 minutes.

4. Add the lemon juice and let cook for a few minutes.

5. Add the kale and place a lid on the pan. Cook for a few minutes or until the kale has wilted.

6. Stir the mixture well and add the mesclun greens. Cook for an additional 2 minutes. Garnish with the currants and serve immediately.

- -

POWER BOOST: *Add white beans for an extra dose of protein.*

TIME SAVER: *Follow steps 1 through 4, and then serve over raw kale and raw mesclun greens.*

MONEY SAVER: *Skip the mesclun greens and just stick to the kale.*

Lentil–Quinoa Burger

6 SERVINGS

BURGERS

> 1 cup (170 g) tri-colored quinoa, rinsed
>
> 5 cups (1.19 L) water, divided
>
> 1 cup (77 g) sprouted green lentils
>
> Spices of your choice, to taste (dried cumin, paprika, dried onion flakes, etc.)

SAUCE

> 1 tomato, chopped
>
> ¼ cup (38 g) red onion, chopped
>
> 2 red chiles
>
> 2 cloves garlic, minced
>
> ½ cup (119 mL) water
>
> ⅓ cup (79 mL) olive oil
>
> 2 tablespoons brown rice vinegar
>
> Lemon juice, to taste

1. In a saucepan, combine the quinoa and 2 cups (474 mL) of the water. Bring to a boil, cover, and lower the heat to medium. Cook for 15 minutes or until the quinoa is done.

2. While the quinoa is cooking, combine all the sauce ingredients, except the lemon juice, in another saucepan. Heat the sauce for 5 minutes and transfer it to a blender. Blend until it is smooth, and season to taste with the lemon juice. Return to the pan and cook it over low heat for 5 minutes, or until it is warm.

3. In a medium saucepan, bring the remaining 3 cups (711 mL) of water to a boil. Pour in the lentils and gently boil for 5 minutes. Remove them from the heat. Cover the lentils and let them stand for 4 to 8 minutes.

4. Combine the quinoa and lentils in a food processor with half of the sauce and any spices you want to use. Pulse until the mixture is well combined, but not too wet.

5. With your hands, shape the mixture into medium-sized patties. Place the patties in the refrigerator for a few minutes to let them set before cooking.

CONTINUED ON NEXT PAGE

6. On a greased griddle or skillet, cook each patty for 5 minutes per side. Cover the patties with the remaining sauce and enjoy!

POWER BOOST: *Serve the burgers over a bed of fresh arugula or wrap them in collard greens for a powerful dose of green veggies.*

TIME SAVER: *Make the patties the night before and refrigerate. The next day, pop them in the oven on a cookie sheet covered in parchment paper and bake them for 20 minutes at 350°F (180°C) or until the desired texture is reached.*

MONEY SAVER: *Instead of purchasing a bag of sprouted green lentils, purchase lentils from a bulk bin, or packaged green lentils.*

Mac and Cheese

*This recipe is adapted from Heather Crosby's **YumUniverse** recipe.*

6 SERVINGS

> **1 box Ancient Harvest Quinoa Gluten Free Elbows pasta (or noodles of your choice)**
>
> **2 cups (276 g) cashews**
>
> **4 cups (474 mL) water**
>
> **½ cup (119 mL) extra virgin coconut oil**
>
> **6 tablespoons (72 g) nutritional yeast**
>
> **6 tablespoons (90 mL) tahini**
>
> **Juice of 2 lemons**

1. Cook the pasta according to the package directions.

2. Combine the remaining ingredients in the blender and blend until smooth.

3. Transfer the mixture from the blender to a saucepan and warm over medium heat, stirring often.

4. Once the pasta has cooked, drain it, combine it with the sauce, and mix until creamy. Serve!

- -

POWER BOOST: *Add fresh veggies to the sauce, such as zucchini, tomato, red pepper, or yellow squash.*

TIME SAVER: *Instead of using pasta, peel zucchini into strips with a vegetable peeler and toss it into the saucepan for a grain-free treat.*

MONEY SAVER: *Look for big tubs of nutritional yeast, often sold in the supplements section of stores. They are often cheaper than buying in smaller quantities (you can get a huge tub at Whole Foods for $8.95).*

Portobello Mushroom Burger

4 SERVINGS

> 4 portobello mushroom caps, stems removed
>
> ¼ cup (59 mL) balsamic vinegar
>
> 2 tablespoons extra virgin olive oil, divided
>
> 1 teaspoon torn fresh basil
>
> 1 teaspoon dried oregano
>
> 2 cloves garlic, minced
>
> Sliced red onion, for topping
>
> Sliced avocado, for topping

1. Place the mushroom caps in a shallow dish with their stem sides down.

2. In a small bowl, whisk together the vinegar, 1 tablespoon of the oil, the basil, the oregano, and the garlic. Pour this mixture over the mushrooms. Marinate the mushrooms for 10 minutes, turning them twice.

3. Heat the remaining oil in a large pan over medium heat. Cook the mushrooms, frequently brushing them with the marinade, for 3 to 5 minutes per side, or until they are tender. Top them with the red onion and avocado and serve.

- -

POWER BOOST: *Serve the burgers over fresh spinach.*

TIME SAVER: *Instead of letting the mushrooms marinate, simply pour the marinade over the mushrooms as they cook.*

MONEY SAVER: *Purchase portobellos loose instead of in packages.*

Power Chili

8 SERVINGS

  2 tablespoons coconut or olive oil

  1 small yellow onion, chopped

  1 large red bell pepper, chopped

  1 large jalapeño pepper, chopped

  4 cloves garlic, chopped

  1 cup (237 mL) pale beer (try Green's gluten-free beers) or low-sodium veggie broth

  3 tomatoes, chopped

  3 15-ounce (426-g) cans or boxes low-sodium red beans, mostly drained

  2 15-ounce (426-g) cans or boxes low-sodium black beans, mostly drained

  2 tablespoons chili powder (or more, to taste)

  1 tablespoon ground cumin

  1 tablespoon ground cayenne

  1 (15-ounce [426-g]) can vegetarian refried beans (look for lower-sodium varieties)

  2 cups (474 mL) water (optional, for cooking quinoa)

  1 cup quinoa (optional)

  Chopped scallions, for topping

  Vegan sour cream, vegan cheese, or nutritional yeast (optional)

1. Pour the oil into a deep, heavy saucepan placed over medium heat. Add the onion, red pepper, jalapeño pepper, and garlic. Sauté for 5 minutes to soften the vegetables.

2. Add the beer or broth, tomatoes, red beans, and black beans. Stir to combine. Add the chili powder, cumin, and cayenne. Thicken the mixture by stirring in the refried beans.

3. Simmer the chili over low heat for 5 to 10 minutes, or longer.

4. If you are using the quinoa, bring the water and the quinoa to a boil. Reduce the heat, cover, and cook for 12 to 15 minutes.

CONTINUED ON NEXT PAGE

5. Once the quinoa is done, stir it into the chili. Serve the chili topped with the scallions and vegan sour cream, vegan cheese, or nutritional yeast.

- -

POWER BOOST: *The night before making chili, soak the quinoa for 10 to 12 hours. In the morning, drain the quinoa and leave it in a bowl with a paper towel draped over the top to sprout. That evening, cook the quinoa with the chili.*

TIME SAVER: *Use dried onion flakes and skip the peppers to avoid chopping.*

MONEY SAVER: *Instead of buying canned refried beans, make your own by mashing black or pinto beans and seasoning them appropriately.*

Raw Bean Salad

4 SERVINGS

>   **6 grape tomatoes, halved**
>
>   **1 carrot, chopped**
>
>   **1 blood orange, peeled and chopped**
>
>   **1 celery stick, chopped**
>
>   **Handful cooked garbanzo beans**
>
>   **Handful walnuts**
>
>   **2 tablespoons apple cider vinegar**
>
>   **2 tablespoons raw pumpkin seeds**
>
>   **Dash salt-free Mexican seasoning (optional)**

1. Toss all the ingredients together and serve!

- -

POWER BOOST: *Cook and add a healthy pseudograin, such as quinoa, for an added dose of fiber, iron, and protein.*

TIME SAVER: *Prepare a larger portion and serve it over greens for a more complete salad that can be divided to eat throughout the week.*

MONEY SAVER: *Purchase seeds and walnuts from bulk bins instead of in individual packages. Look for raw options.*

Raw Watermelon and Tomato Salad

4 SERVINGS

>   **2 handfuls cubed watermelon**
>
>   **Handful cherry or grape tomatoes, cut in half**
>
>   **¼ red onion, cut into slivers**
>
>   **3 large basil leaves, roughly chopped or torn**
>
>   **Balsamic vinegar, for drizzling**

1. Toss all the ingredients together in a medium bowl and drizzle with balsamic vinegar. Serve.

- -

POWER BOOST: *Toss pumpkin seeds into the salad for an extra dose of iron.*

TIME SAVER: *Purchase sliced watermelon if you don't have time to slice an entire watermelon (though purchasing a whole watermelon is cheaper and will make more).*

MONEY SAVER: *Look for fresh bunches of basil instead of prepackaged basil, which can be almost triple the cost of the loose-leaf variety.*

Red Bean Burger

6 SERVINGS

2 (15-ounce [426-g]) cans or boxes low-sodium red beans, drained and rinsed

¼ cup (38 g) plus 2 tablespoons bread crumbs

¼ cup (6 g) chopped cilantro

1 clove garlic, minced

1 flax egg or chia egg (mix 2 tablespoons ground flax or chia seeds with 3 tablespoons [45 mL] water, and refrigerate for a few minutes)

1 teaspoon chili powder

1 teaspoon ground coriander

1 teaspoon ground cumin

Freshly ground black pepper, to taste

Coconut oil, for cooking

Lettuce, avocado, and tomato, for topping (optional)

1. Place all the ingredients, except the coconut oil and toppings, in a food processor. Process the ingredients until well combined, but not overly processed.

2. Form the mixture into small round patties.

3. Using a griddle or skillet, heat the coconut oil over medium heat. Cook the patties until they are sizzling and lightly browned. Flip them and cook an additional few minutes. Add the toppings and serve.

- -

POWER BOOST: *Mix sacha inchi or hemp seeds into the burgers.*

TIME SAVER: *Double the recipe and freeze it (before cooking) until ready to heat and eat.*

MONEY SAVER: *Skip the toppings and bake the burgers, so you don't have to use (or purchase) oil.*

Squash–Sunflower Seed Soup

6 SERVINGS

- **1 tablespoon olive or coconut oil**
- **1 medium onion, chopped (about 2 cups [300 g])**
- **1 tablespoon grated ginger**
- **½ teaspoon ground cayenne**
- **2 large carrots, chopped (about 1 cup [128 g])**
- **1 or 2 large yellow summer squash, peeled and chopped (about 2 cups [226 g])**
- **4 cups (948 mL) low-sodium vegetable stock or water**
- **Pumpkin seeds, for garnish (optional)**
- **2 cups (474 mL) low-sodium tomato juice**
- **1 cup (237 mL) natural sunflower seed butter**
- **½ cup (24 g) chopped chives, for garnish**

1. In a large, heavy saucepan, heat the oil over medium-high heat. Add the onion and sauté until it is translucent.

2. Stir in the ginger and cayenne. Cook them for 1 minute, then add the carrots and sauté a couple more minutes.

3. Add the squash and stock. Bring to a boil and then simmer for about 15 minutes, or until the vegetables are tender.

4. While the vegetables are simmering, toast the pumpkin seeds in a dry pan on low heat for 4 or 5 minutes until they have browned (if using).

5. In a blender or food processor, pureé the vegetables and stock with the cooking liquid and tomato juice.

6. Return the soup to the saucepan. Stir in the sunflower seed butter until smooth. Garnish with the chives and toasted pumpkin seeds and serve.

- -

POWER BOOST: *If you want a more savory soup with a big dose of vitamin A, add a bit of canned pumpkin.*

TIME SAVER: *Top the soup with fresh pumpkin seeds instead of toasted.*

MONEY SAVER: *Make your own sunflower seed butter by grinding sunflower seeds.*

Sweet Potato Fries

4 SERVINGS

   2 or 3 large sweet potatoes, peeled, halved, and cut into steak fries

   3 cloves garlic, chopped

   ¼ cup (8 g) chopped fresh parsley

   ¼ cup (32 g) pumpkin seeds

   2 tablespoons dried oregano

   2 tablespoons paprika

   1 teaspoon ground cayenne

   2 tablespoons coconut oil, melted, or extra virgin olive oil

1. Preheat the oven to 350°F (180°C).

2. In a large bowl, combine the sweet potatoes with the garlic, parsley, pumpkin seeds, oregano, and spices. Toss with the oil.

3. Arrange the sweet potatoes on a baking sheet lined with parchment paper, and bake them until they are tender and golden, 30 to 40 minutes. Serve.

- -

POWER BOOST: *Toss sesame seeds with the sweet potatoes before baking.*

TIME SAVER: *Bump up the oven temperature for quicker cooking (though vitamins and minerals are best maintained at lower oven temperatures).*

MONEY SAVER: *Purchase spices from bulk bins or containers, rather than in individual glass containers.*

Tomato, White Bean, and Spinach Soup

4 SERVINGS

> 1 teaspoon coconut oil
>
> 2 broccoli stalks, chopped
>
> 2 cups (474 mL) water
>
> 2 tomatoes, cut in half
>
> 2 cloves garlic
>
> 1 red bell pepper, chopped
>
> 2 dashes salt-free Mexican seasoning
>
> Juice of 1 lemon
>
> 1 tablespoon Bragg's Liquid Aminos
>
> ½ cup (89 g) cooked white beans
>
> Handful spinach

1. In a saucepan, heat the coconut oil over medium heat. Add all the ingredients except the beans and spinach. Cook for 5 minutes, stirring often.

2. Place the contents of the saucepan in a blender. Blend and return to the pan. Add the white beans and spinach. Serve!

- -

POWER BOOST: *Add a healthy grain for a heartier, longer-lasting meal.*

TIME SAVER: *Throw the soup over pasta the next night for a delicious dinner!*

MONEY SAVER: *Purchase frozen spinach instead of fresh.*

Veggie Pizza

1 PIZZA

>2 tablespoons olive oil, divided
>
>1 beet, cleaned
>
>1 acorn squash, halved
>
>7 homegrown tomatoes
>
>1 bunch fresh basil
>
>1 bunch fresh oregano
>
>⅓ cup (48 g) almonds
>
>3 cloves garlic, minced
>
>1 bunch garlic chives, minced
>
>½ leek, thinly sliced
>
>Juice of 1 lemon
>
>1 bunch kale, finely chopped
>
>1 bunch mesclun greens
>
>2 (7-ounce [200-g]) jars organic low-sodium tomato paste
>
>1 organic pizza crust
>
>1 bell pepper, chopped
>
>Handful white button mushrooms, sliced
>
>1 (8-ounce [227-g]) package Daiya Mozzarella Style Shreds

1. Preheat the oven to 400°F (200°C). With a paper towel or brush, rub inside the squash with a dab of olive oil. Place the beet and the acorn squash in a baking pan to roast. Roast both until they are tender (about 20 minutes). Once they are done, remove them from the oven. Let them sit while you prepare the other ingredients. Once the beet is cool, remove its skin and slice. Remove the rind from the acorn squash and slice.

2. Cut 5 of the tomatoes in half. Place the basil on the bottom of a small baking pan. Lay the halved tomatoes on the basil, and top them with the fresh oregano. Cover with the aluminum foil and heat in the oven for about 15 minutes.

3. Make a garlic chive pesto by toasting the almonds in a dry pan for 5 minutes. Place the almonds, garlic, garlic chives, and 1 tablespoon of the olive oil in a food processor. Process these ingredients until they are well combined.

CONTINUED ON NEXT PAGE

4. In a sauté pan, combine the remaining tablespoon of olive oil, the leek, and two heaping spoonfuls of the pesto. Cook these over medium heat for 1 to 2 minutes. Add the lemon juice and let cook for a few more minutes. Add the kale and place a lid on the pan. Cook for a few minutes or until the kale has wilted.

5. Stir the mixture well and add the mesclun greens. Cook for an additional 2 minutes. Set aside.

6. Once the tomatoes, basil, and oregano have come out of the oven, place them in a saucepan over high heat and let them cook down for about 10 minutes to make a sauce (they should start to thicken). Stir in the tomato paste and a spoonful of pesto. Let the sauce simmer until the pizza is ready to assemble.

7. Slice the remaining 2 tomatoes.

8. On the crust, layer the tomato sauce, the kale and pesto mixture, the acorn squash, the beet, the bell pepper, and the mushrooms. Sprinkle the Daiya Mozzarella Style Shreds on top.

9. Bake the pizza for 12 minutes, or until the crust is tender. Serve.

- -

POWER BOOST: *Instead of using Daiya Mozzarella Style Shreds, sprinkle nutritional yeast on top of the pizza.*

TIME SAVER: *Don't roast the vegetables or make your own tomato sauce or pesto. Use tomato paste as the sauce. Place raw vegetables on the crust, and bake.*

MONEY SAVER: *Skip the tomato paste and just blend the tomatoes to make a sauce.*

Zucchini Pasta with Tomato Sauce

6 SERVINGS

TOMATO SAUCE

1–2 tablespoons extra virgin olive oil

1–2 tablespoons water

⅓ cup (50 g) diced white onion

4 garlic cloves, minced

Paprika, ground cayenne, and dried oregano, to taste

8 vine-ripened tomatoes, chopped

⅓ cup (79 mL) red wine (optional)

1–2 (7-ounce [200-g]) jars organic low-sodium

½ red bell pepper, diced

⅓ cup (8 g) fresh basil, chopped

ZUCCHINI PASTA

1–2 tablespoons extra virgin olive oil

4–5 zucchini, sliced into strips with a vegetable peeler

1. In a large pan, heat 1 to 2 tablespoons of oil. Add the water, onion, garlic, paprika, cayenne, and oregano, and sauté until the onion is just tender.

2. Add the tomatoes and the red wine to the pan. Cover the pan and let the sauce simmer for 10 to 12 minutes, or until the tomatoes start to reduce.

3. Once the tomatoes have reduced, add the tomato paste, stirring frequently. Add the bell pepper and continue cooking. Once the bell pepper softens, reduce the heat to low and add the basil.

4. In another pan, heat 1 to 2 tablespoons of oil. Drop the zucchini strips into the pan. Sauté them for 2 to 3 minutes or longer. Top the zucchini strips with the sauce and serve.

- -

POWER BOOST: *Top the dish with nutritional yeast.*

TIME SAVER: *Instead of cooking the zucchini separately, toss it directly into the sauce when the sauce is almost done cooking.*

MONEY SAVER: *Purchase regular organic tomatoes instead of vine-ripened tomatoes when making your own sauce.*

Sweet Recipes

Almond and Sunflower Seed Granola

4 SERVINGS

> **3 tablespoons (30 mL) coconut oil**
>
> **2 heaping tablespoons honey, agave nectar, or molasses**
>
> **2 cups (162 g) old-fashioned oats**
>
> **½ cup (72 g) raw almonds**
>
> **⅓ cup (15 g) sunflower seeds**
>
> **Ground cinnamon, to taste**
>
> **Sea salt, to taste (optional)**

1. Preheat the oven to 325°F (160°C). Line a cookie sheet with parchment paper.

2. In a small pan, combine the coconut oil and honey. Bring them to a simmer over medium heat, stirring constantly until the coconut oil turns to liquid (about 2 minutes).

3. In a bowl, combine the oats, almonds, and sunflower seeds. Season to taste with the cinnamon and the sea salt (if using). Pour the oil and honey mixture over the dry ingredients and stir to coat the dry ingredients evenly.

4. Spread the mixture onto the prepared cookie sheet and bake it for 20 minutes, stirring halfway through the baking time.

5. Remove the granola from the oven and let it cool. Serve on its own or with nondairy milk and berries.

- -

POWER BOOST: *Add dried fruit or different seeds to the recipe for a nutrition boost.*

TIME SAVER: *Make a large batch of granola that will last the entire week. Store in a glass container on the counter so you can have your cereal every morning, or take it to work as a healthy "trail mix" snack.*

MONEY SAVER: *Purchase oats from bulk bins, which can save over $5 per serving!*

Almond Milk and Apricot Muesli

2 SERVINGS

> 1 cup (81 g) old-fashioned oats
>
> Almond milk (enough to cover oats)
>
> 2 tablespoons chopped dried apricots
>
> 1 tablespoon flax seeds
>
> 1 tablespoon hemp seed butter
>
> 1 teaspoon honey or agave nectar (or more, to taste)
>
> Ground cinnamon, to taste

1. Place the oats in a small- to medium-sized glass bowl with a lid. Pour the almond milk on top of the oats until they are well covered. Snap the lid on.

2. Place the bowl in the refrigerator overnight.

3. In the morning, remove the lid and stir the oats. Add the apricots, flax seeds, and hemp seed butter, stirring well. Season to taste with the honey or agave nectar and the cinnamon. Serve the muesli cold.

- -

POWER BOOST: *Purchase sprouted flax seeds for optimal nutrition, or sprout them yourself (see page 58).*

TIME SAVER: *Double or triple the recipe so you have two or three days' worth of breakfasts that you can grab and go.*

MONEY SAVER: *Rather than invest in hemp seed butter (which can run around $30 per container), grind hemp seeds yourself, or opt for a more inexpensive butter, like almond or cashew.*

Apple Almond Butter Sandwich

4 SERVINGS

2 red apples, sliced into 8 thick, horizontal pieces (to resemble bread)

2 tablespoons almond butter

1 teaspoon chia seeds

1 tablespoon raisins

1 banana, sliced

1. Spread the almond butter on the apple slices. Sprinkle the chia seeds and raisins on the slices, and place the bananas on the apple slices. Press the slices together to make 4 sandwiches and serve.

- -

POWER BOOST: *Purchase raw, sprouted almond butter.*

TIME SAVER: *Make a big batch and store in the refrigerator to have snacks on hand (kids love them).*

MONEY SAVER: *Make your own almond butter by grinding almonds.*

Banana–Walnut–Chocolate Bread

1 8X4-INCH (20X10-CM) LOAF

> **½ cup (119 mL) coconut oil, room temperature, plus more to grease loaf pan**
>
> **2 cups (250 g) spelt flour (or a gluten-free baking flour of your choice)**
>
> **½ teaspoon baking soda**
>
> **1 teaspoon ground cinnamon**
>
> **¾ cup (166 g) coconut palm sugar or Sucanat**
>
> **3 very ripe bananas, mashed well with a fork**
>
> **¼ cup (59 mL) nondairy milk, mixed with 1 teaspoon apple cider vinegar**
>
> **½ cup (50 g) walnuts**
>
> **Vegan chocolate chips (optional)**

1. Preheat the oven to 300°F (150°C). Grease an 8x4-inch (20x10-cm) loaf pan with coconut oil.

2. In a medium bowl, sift together the flour, baking soda, and cinnamon.

3. In a food processor, process the remaining ½ cup of coconut oil and the sugar. Add the bananas and milk mixture, and process.

4. Pour the wet ingredients from the food processor into the dry ingredients and mix them well.

5. Fold in the walnuts and the chocolate chips (if using).

6. Pour the batter into the prepared loaf pan. Bake for 55 minutes, or until a toothpick inserted in the center of the bread comes out clean. Let cool, then serve.

- -

POWER BOOST: *Use raw walnuts for a good dose of Omega-3s.*

TIME SAVER: *Make muffins instead of bread and bake them for just 20 minutes.*

MONEY SAVER: *Purchase conventional bananas.*

Blueberry Oat Bar

15 BARS

> **1½ cups (221 g) pitted dates**
> **⅓ cup (27 g) old-fashioned rolled oats**
> **½ cup (73 g) blueberries**
> **¼ cup (34 g) raw macadamia nuts**

1. Pulse all the ingredients in a food processor until they are combined.

2. Press the mixture into the bottom of a glass container or 9x5-inch (22.5x12.5-cm) loaf pan.

3. Slice the mixture into rectangular bars and serve.

> **COOKS' NOTE: Store the extra bars in the refrigerator.**

- -

POWER BOOST: *Vary your berries for added antioxidants.*

TIME SAVER: *Buy pitted dates to save you time pitting them at home.*

MONEY SAVER: *Try a different type of nut, as macadamias can be expensive.*

Cashew–Chocolate Chip–Oatmeal Cookies

12–15 COOKIES

> **1 cup (138 g) raw cashews**
>
> **Splash nondairy milk**
>
> **½ banana, mashed**
>
> **½ cup (41 g) oats**
>
> **⅓ cup (74 g) coconut palm sugar or Sucanat**
>
> **½ cup (90 g) vegan chocolate chips**
>
> **1 flax egg or chia egg (mix 2 tablespoons ground flax or chia seeds with 3 tablespoons [45 mL] water, and refrigerate for a few minutes)**
>
> **1 teaspoon baking powder**
>
> **½ teaspoon baking soda**

1. Preheat the oven to 350°F (180°C). Line a cookie sheet with parchment paper.

2. Process the cashews in a food processor until they are crushed. With the power still on, dribble in the nondairy milk to help soften the cashews. (They will lump together and become pastelike.)

3. In a large bowl, combine the cashew mixture with all the remaining ingredients, stirring well. Gauge the consistency and taste to see if you want more or less chocolate, oats, or sugar.

4. Spoon the mixture into small rounds on the prepared cookie sheet and slightly flatten them into discs (the batter will be sticky).

5. Bake the cookies for 8 to 10 minutes. Remove them, let them cool, and then serve. (These cookies do not spread like regular cookies. Look for a slightly browned top to know that they are done. They will firm up once they are cool.)

- -

POWER BOOST: *If you have a dehydrator, make the mixture sans baking powder and baking soda and dehydrate for a raw cookie.*

TIME SAVER: *Instead of blending the cashews, opt for 1 cup (237 mL) of almond, cashew, or peanut butter.*

MONEY SAVER: *Make a giant batch of cookies to have on hand for the week. When sweet cravings strike, you won't opt for buying that muffin or cookie out, which costs much more.*

Chocolate Beet Cake

1 8-INCH (20-CM) CAKE

>   ¼ cup (59 mL) coconut oil, room temperature, plus more to grease baking pan
>
>   1 beet, peeled and diced
>
>   1 cup (237 mL) almond milk (or nondairy milk of your choice)
>
>   1 banana
>
>   ½ cup (43 g) cocoa or cacao powder
>
>   ⅓ cup (74 g) coconut palm sugar or Sucanat
>
>   1 teaspoon vanilla extract
>
>   1¾ cup (295 g) spelt flour (or a gluten-free baking flour of your choice)
>
>   2 teaspoons baking powder
>
>   ½ cup (50 g) walnuts (optional)

1. Preheat the oven to 350°F (180°C). Grease an 8-inch (20-cm) baking pan with coconut oil.

2. While the oven is preheating, steam the beet on the stovetop until it can be easily pierced with a fork. Once the beet is done, pureé it in a food processor with the milk, banana, cocoa or cacao powder, sugar, and vanilla extract.

3. Sift the flour and baking powder together in a bowl.

4. Fold the wet ingredients into the dry, and stir in the walnuts (if using).

5. Pour the batter into the prepared baking pan and bake for 30 minutes, or until a toothpick inserted in the center of the cake comes out clean. Let cool, then serve.

- -

POWER BOOST: *Add a tablespoon of apple cider vinegar to the wet ingredients.*

TIME SAVER: *Microwave the beet until it is soft, and then dice.*

MONEY SAVER: *Use raw sugar instead of Sucanat.*

Chocolate Chip Blueberry Pancakes

6 PANCAKES

> 1 tablespoon apple cider vinegar
>
> 1 cup (237 mL) nondairy milk
>
> 1 flax egg or chia egg (mix 2 tablespoons ground flax or chia seeds with 3 tablespoons [45 mL] water, and refrigerate for a few minutes)
>
> ½ cup (113 g) mashed banana
>
> 1 cup (130 g) buckwheat flour or oat flour
>
> 1 teaspoon baking powder
>
> ¼ teaspoon baking soda
>
> 2 heaping tablespoons cocoa or cacao powder
>
> 1 tablespoon ground cinnamon
>
> ½ cup (73 g) blueberries (optional)
>
> ½ cup (50 g) walnuts (optional)
>
> ½ cup (90 g) vegan chocolate chips (optional)
>
> Agave nectar or raw honey, for topping

1. Combine the apple cider vinegar and nondairy milk in a bowl and let the mixture curdle like buttermilk.

2. Add the flax egg and mashed banana to the "buttermilk" mixture and whisk them together until smooth.

3. In a separate bowl, mix the flour, baking powder, baking soda, cocoa, and cinnamon. Create a well in the center of the flour mixture, and pour in the wet ingredients. Stir.

4. Fold in the blueberries, walnuts, and chocolate chips, if using. Mix until there are very few lumps.

5. Heat a skillet or griddle rubbed lightly with coconut oil over medium heat.

6. Spoon about 1/6 of the batter onto the prepared skillet, and cook until the edges begin to lift and the uncooked side is bubbly. Flip the pancake and cook it for an additional couple of minutes, then remove it from the heat. Repeat this step with the remaining batter.

7. Serve the pancakes topped with the agave nectar or raw honey and more fresh berries!

CONTINUED ON NEXT PAGE

- -

POWER BOOST: *Sprinkle the tops of the pancakes with hemp or chia seeds.*

TIME SAVER: *Double or triple the recipe and make a large batch to have on hand for snacks or an after-dinner treat.*

MONEY SAVER: *Rather than investing in nondairy milk, make your own by grinding seeds or nuts with water in a blender and then straining through a mesh strainer or nut bag. Grind oats to make your own oat flour instead of purchasing oat or buckwheat flour.*

Chocolate Greens Smoothie

1–2 SERVINGS

Handful baby spinach or kale

1 cup (155 g) frozen blueberries

½ cup (111 g) frozen strawberries

½ cup (119 mL) unsweetened almond milk (or nondairy milk of your choice)

1 banana

2 tablespoons cocoa or cacao powder

2 Medjool dates, pitted

1 tablespoon ground flax

1. Blend all the ingredients until smooth, and serve!

- -

POWER BOOST: *Add a scoop of wheatgrass powder to the smoothie.*

TIME SAVER: *Buy 1 or 2 bunches of bananas, peel them, and pop them in a Ziploc bag. Store them in the freezer and use them for smoothies (you can forgo ice when you use this method). This makes for a much creamier smoothie!*

MONEY SAVER: *Try Deglet dates instead of Medjool, which are more expensive. Search the bulk bin section of your grocery store.*

Chocolate Ice Cream

*This recipe is adapted from Heather Crosby's **YumUniverse** recipe.*

4 SERVINGS

10 dates, pitted and chopped

2 cups (474 mL) water or nondairy milk

¼ cup cocoa or cacao powder

2 tablespoons almond butter (or other nut butter)

1 teaspoon vanilla extract

Walnuts, for topping (optional)

Strawberries, for topping (optional)

1. Toss all the ingredients, except the toppings, in a blender. Blend for several minutes until completely smooth and creamy.

2. Pour the mixture into a glass container and let it sit in the freezer, uncovered, until it is frozen. (Time can vary from 1 to 4 hours.)

3. Serve the ice cream topped with the walnuts and fresh berries!

> **COOKS' NOTE: Have an ice cream maker? Instead of freezing, pop the mixture in the freezer at step 2 for 5 to 10 minutes and then follow the ice cream maker's instructions.**

- -

POWER BOOST: *Replace the cocoa or cacao powder with chocolate hemp protein powder.*

TIME SAVER: *Double or triple the recipe and store in the freezer so you have enough for the entire week.*

MONEY SAVER: *Purchase regular cocoa instead of raw cacao, which can be expensive.*

Chocolate Pumpkin Pudding

4 SERVINGS

3 avocados, pitted

½ cup (123 g) canned pure pumpkin

¼ cup (59 mL) raw agave nectar or raw honey

6 tablespoons (32 g) cocoa or cacao powder

1 teaspoon vanilla extract (optional)

Fresh berries, for topping (optional)

1. Place all the ingredients, except the berries, in a food processor. Blend them until the mixture is smooth.

2. Place the mixture in the refrigerator until it is cold. Top with the fresh berries and enjoy.

- -

POWER BOOST: *Add chia or hemp seeds before processing.*

TIME SAVER: *Blend the pudding in the morning and place it in an airtight container in the refrigerator, so you will have it on hand when you get home later that day.*

MONEY SAVER: *Purchase conventional avocados.*

Dark Chocolate, Chia, and Cherry Pecan Bar

8 PIECES

2 bars dark chocolate (70 percent dark) or vegan chocolate

Vegetable oil spray

½ cup (50 g) raw pecans, chopped

⅓ cup (37 g) unsweetened dried cherries

1 tablespoon chia seeds

Dash sea salt

1. Melt the chocolate over medium heat in a double boiler, breaking the chocolate apart and stirring it frequently. (If you don't have a double boiler, fill a saucepan partway with water, place the chocolate in a heat-safe glass bowl on top of it, and heat until the chocolate is melted.)

2. Grease an 8-inch (20-cm) baking dish with the vegetable oil spray, then line it with parchment paper, allowing a slight overhang.

3. Once the chocolate is melted, pour it into the prepared baking dish.

4. Sprinkle the pecans, cherries, and chia seeds on top of the chocolate, add the sea salt, and chill the chocolate in the refrigerator for 30 minutes, until set.

5. When you want to serve the bars, peel the chocolate off of the parchment paper and break it into pieces.

- -

POWER BOOST: *Add chopped walnuts, pistachios, or sprouted uncooked quinoa for added fiber, protein, iron, and an Omega-3 boost.*

TIME SAVER: *Melt the chocolate in the microwave instead.*

MONEY SAVER: *Look for loose chocolate chips in bulk bins instead of purchasing bars of chocolate, which can cost more.*

Green Superfood Energy Bar

10 BARS

> **20 dates, pitted**
>
> **½ cup (65 g) raw pumpkin seeds**
>
> **½ cup (76 g) raw pistachios**
>
> **½ cup (65 g) hemp seeds**
>
> **1 tablespoon spirulina**
>
> **Juice of 1 lime**

1. In a food processor, process all the ingredients until they are well combined.

2. Press the mixture into a glass container, or spread it on a cutting board. Cover the mixture with plastic wrap or parchment paper and roll flat with a rolling pin. Remove the wrap or paper, cut the mixture into bars, and serve.

> **COOKS' NOTE: Store the bars in individual plastic bags or wrap them in parchment paper. (You can store the bars in the freezer or refrigerator and take them out as needed.)**

- -

POWER BOOST: *Add a tablespoon of wheatgrass powder or chlorella to the recipe.*

TIME SAVER: *Double the recipe and store the bars in the refrigerator or freezer so you have easy, portable snacks for the entire week.*

MONEY SAVER: *Purchase all seeds and nuts in bulk from online retailers once per month. Sunfood (sunfood.com) offers good deals.*

Chocolate–Hazelnut Spread

1 CUP (200 G)

1 cup (142 g) hazelnuts, skins removed

2 heaping tablespoons cocoa or cacao powder

2 tablespoons coconut palm sugar or Sucanat

2–4 tablespoons light coconut milk, divided

½ teaspoon vanilla extract

1. In a food processor, blend the hazelnuts for 2 to 3 minutes. They will become warm and almost start to liquefy.

2. Add the cocoa, sugar, and 2 tablespoons of the coconut milk to the food processor. Process until the mixture forms a single, large clump.

3. Remove the mixture from the food processor and vigorously stir in 1 to 2 additional tablespoons of coconut milk, until spread reaches the desired consistency. Serve immediately by spreading on fruit or a slice of bread.

> **COOKS' NOTE: Store leftover spread in an airtight container in the refrigerator.**

- -

POWER BOOST: *Use coconut milk from a fresh coconut instead of a can.*

TIME SAVER: *Buy hazelnuts without their skins.*

MONEY SAVER: *Use a fresh vanilla bean instead of purchasing vanilla extract.*

Peanut Butter Smoothie

1–2 SERVINGS

> **5 ice cubes**
>
> **½ cup (119 mL) nondairy milk**
>
> **1 banana**
>
> **1 scoop hemp, pea, or brown rice protein**
>
> **2 tablespoons natural peanut butter (or nut butter of your choice)**
>
> **1 teaspoon cocoa or cacao powder**
>
> **Ground cinnamon, to taste**

1. In a blender, combine the ice cubes, nondairy milk, and banana. Gradually add the hemp protein, peanut butter, and cocoa. Blend the ingredients until they are well combined. Season to taste with the cinnamon. Serve!

- -

POWER BOOST: *Sprinkle in some sacha inchi seeds.*

TIME SAVER: *Store jars of nut butters upside down so that the oil naturally mixes. When you open the jar, voila! No spending minutes at a time trying to stir an oily mess.*

MONEY SAVER: *Make your own nut butters by grinding nuts in a food processor. You can add oil, sea salt, and agave nectar or honey as you prefer.*

Pineapple Almond Poppers

This recipe is adapted from Jenné Claiborne's recipe from Sweet Potato Soul.

16 POPPERS

> **1 cup (143 g) almonds**
> **1 cup (112 g) dried pineapple, diced**
> **½ cup (74 g) dates, diced**
> **4 dried apricots, diced**
> **½ teaspoon ground cinnamon**
> **1 tablespoon coconut oil**
> **¼ teaspoon vanilla extract**
> **Juice of 1 lemon**
> **½ cup (40 g) shredded coconut**

1. In a food processor, grind the almonds to a fine meal.

2. Add the pineapple, dates, apricots, and cinnamon to the food processor and process until well combined.

3. Pour in the coconut oil and vanilla extract and process the mixture for a few seconds. Add the lemon juice.

4. Taste the mixture and add more fruit, spice, or oil if necessary. The consistency should be a bit chunky and should hold together when formed.

5. Form the dough into small or large balls, and roll them in the shredded coconut to coat.

6. Place the balls on a plate to chill in the refrigerator for at least 30 minutes before you enjoy them.

- -

POWER BOOST: *Add hemp seeds to the mixture.*

TIME SAVER: *Press the mixture flat and cut it into bars instead of rolling it into balls. Sprinkle the coconut on top.*

MONEY SAVER: *Purchase loose, dried fruit instead of prepackaged whenever possible. Or dehydrate your own fruit in the oven!*

Pumpkin Pie Smoothie

1–2 SERVINGS

> **5 ice cubes**
>
> **½ cup (119 mL) soy, almond, or hemp milk**
>
> **1 banana**
>
> **½ cup (123 g) canned pure pumpkin**
>
> **1 teaspoon ground cinnamon**
>
> **1 scoop hemp, pea, or brown rice protein**

1. In a blender, combine the ice cubes, milk, and banana. Blend them, and then gradually add the pumpkin, cinnamon, and hemp protein. Serve.

- -

POWER BOOST: *If time allows, use fresh baked pumpkin instead of canned.*

TIME SAVER: *Make the smoothie first thing in the morning and place it in the freezer to let it chill a bit before you drink it, so it's more like a milkshake.*

MONEY SAVER: *Compare hemp protein to brown rice or pea protein to see which gives you the best bang for your buck.*

Quinoa with Fruit and Nuts

2 SERVINGS

1 cup (170 g) quinoa, rinsed, uncooked

2 cups (474 mL) water

½ cup (73 g) blueberries

⅓ cup (37 g) dried cranberries

½ teaspoon ground cinnamon

⅓ cup (33 g) walnuts

1. Add the quinoa to the water in a medium saucepan and bring to a boil. Reduce the heat and simmer for 5 minutes.

2. Add the blueberries, cranberries, and cinnamon to the quinoa. Simmer until all the water has absorbed.

3. Toss in the walnuts and top with the nondairy milk of your choice. Drizzle the quinoa with agave nectar, if desired, and serve.

- -

POWER BOOST: *Use sprouted quinoa (available in most stores, or you can sprout your own).*

TIME SAVER: *Instead of water, use nondairy milk to cook the quinoa.*

MONEY SAVER: *Always purchase quinoa from bulk bins instead of purchasing individual bags, as they can be more than twice the cost.*

Quinoa–Cranberry–Walnut Muffins

12 MUFFINS

Coconut oil to grease muffin tin, if you are not using paper liners

1 cup (135 g) spelt flour (or gluten-free baking flour of your choice)

⅔ cup (148 g) coconut palm sugar or Sucanat

1 tablespoon baking powder

1 teaspoon ground cinnamon

½ teaspoon baking soda

½ teaspoon ground ginger

¼ teaspoon ground nutmeg

1 cup (237 mL) creamy natural cashew butter (or nut butter of your choice)

⅔ cup (158 mL) plus 2 tablespoons nondairy milk

2 teaspoons vanilla extract

⅔ cup (123 g) cooked and cooled quinoa

½ cup (55 g) dried cranberries

⅓ cup (33 g) walnuts

1. Preheat the oven to 350°F (180°C). Line a standard muffin tin with paper liners, or grease it lightly with coconut oil.

2. In a large bowl, whisk together the flour, sugar, baking powder, cinnamon, baking soda, ginger, and nutmeg.

3. In a medium bowl, whisk together the cashew butter, nondairy milk, and vanilla extract.

4. Fold the wet ingredients into the dry, being careful not to overmix.

5. Fold in the quinoa, cranberries, and walnuts.

6. Divide the batter equally among the prepared muffin cups and bake for 20 minutes, or until a toothpick inserted in the center of a muffin comes out clean. Let the muffins cool on a wire rack, and serve.

- -

POWER BOOST: *Use unsweetened or fresh cranberries whenever possible to up the antioxidants and cut sugar.*

TIME SAVER: *Make a big batch of quinoa the night before and simply scoop it into the recipe before baking.*

MONEY SAVER: *Purchase flour from bulk bins instead of in bags whenever possible.*

Strawberry–Oatmeal Smoothie

1–2 SERVINGS

>   **5 ice cubes**
>
>   **⅓ cup (79 mL) almond, soy or hemp milk**
>
>   **½ banana**
>
>   **3–4 strawberries**
>
>   **1 teaspoon ground cinnamon**
>
>   **½ teaspoon ground nutmeg**
>
>   **⅓ cup (78 g) cooked oatmeal**
>
>   **1 scoop hemp, pea, or brown rice protein**

1. In a blender, combine the ice cubes, milk, banana, and strawberries, and blend. Gradually add the cinnamon, nutmeg, oatmeal, and hemp protein. Serve.

- -

POWER BOOST: *Toss in a handful of blueberries for an added antioxidant dose.*

TIME SAVER: *Pour the milk in the blender first (before the ice cubes) to avoid maniacally shaking the blender as you try to mix everything. This can save minutes of yelling at an inanimate object.*

MONEY SAVER: *Purchase frozen strawberries instead of fresh.*

CHAPTER 14

Your Four-Seasons Eating Plan

"Don't dig your grave with your own knife and fork."

—*ENGLISH PROVERB*

Sometimes it's not enough to have recipes or to know generally what to eat—you want to be told what to eat and when.

Using the recipes in this book, I am going to provide four easy meal plans consisting of three days' worth of food for the week (as many of us eat out a few times per week). Each day has three meals with one snack, and the third day has a dessert as well. If you want another snack (to boost your meals to five per day), choose something simple, like organic fruit, nuts, or seeds, a green juice, or a warm soup.

Each week in my meal plan represents a season of the year, so you can get an idea of the seasonal foods your body needs during specific months. These plans are designed around a variety of plants, so you can benefit from various nutrients throughout your day.

This chapter also includes a grocery list of staple foods to have on hand. This list includes all of the supplies needed for these recipes. You can use these lists as a starting point and swap, make concessions, or replace any meal with something you'd prefer. Use the meal plans as general guidelines for creating your own meal plan.

Pay attention to how you feel on specific days and try to chart your progress. Love a particular meal? Figure out how to use those ingredients to make something different, or add them to one of your favorite dishes. Experimentation is the key!

Fall Meal Plan

DAY ONE

MEAL ONE: Pumpkin Pie Smoothie (page 237)

MEAL TWO: Apple Almond Butter Sandwich (page 222)

MEAL THREE: Red Bean Burger with Sweet Potato Fries (page 213 and page 215)

SNACK: Kale and Garlic Chive Pesto Salad (page 204)

DAY TWO

MEAL ONE: Quinoa–Cranberry–Walnut Muffins (page 239)

MEAL TWO: Kale and Sweet Potato Hash (page 203)

MEAL THREE: Squash–Sunflower Seed Soup (page 214)

SNACK: Basil Hummus (page 195)

DAY THREE

MEAL ONE: Kale and Sweet Potato Hash (leftovers from yesterday's lunch)

MEAL TWO: Black Bean Bowl (page 194)

MEAL THREE: Lentil–Quinoa Burger over greens (page 205)

SNACK: Sweet Potato Fries (page 215)

DESSERT: Banana–Walnut–Chocolate Bread (page 223)

Winter Meal Plan

DAY ONE

MEAL ONE: Chocolate Chip Blueberry Pancakes (page 227)

MEAL TWO: Kale and Garlic Chive Pesto Salad (page 204)

MEAL THREE: Mac and Cheese (page 207)

SNACK: Green Superfood Energy Bar (page 233)

DAY TWO

MEAL ONE: Almond and Sunflower Seed Granola (page 220)

MEAL TWO: Portobello Mushroom Burger with leftover kale salad (page 208)

MEAL THREE: Power Chili (page 209)

SNACK: Dark Chocolate, Chia, and Cherry Pecan Bar (page 232)

DAY THREE

MEAL ONE: Blueberry Oat Bar (page 224)

MEAL TWO: Black Bean Quesadillas (page 196)

MEAL THREE: Coconut Curry Vegetable Soup (page 200)

SNACK: Chocolate Chip Blueberry Pancakes (page 227)

DESSERT: Cashew–Chocolate Chip–Oatmeal Cookies (page 225)

Spring Meal Plan

DAY ONE

MEAL ONE: Almond Milk and Apricot Muesli (page 221)

MEAL TWO: Chopped Salad with Dijon Dressing (page 198)

MEAL THREE: Collard Enchiladas (page 201)

SNACK: Blueberry Oat Bar (page 224)

DAY TWO

MEAL ONE: Strawberry–Oatmeal Smoothie (page 240)

MEAL TWO: Citrus Gazpacho (page 199)

MEAL THREE: Veggie Pizza (page 217)

SNACK: Chocolate Greens Smoothie (page 229)

DAY THREE

MEAL ONE: Green Superfood Energy Bar (page 233)

MEAL TWO: Raw Bean Salad (page 211)

MEAL THREE: Tomato, White Bean, and Spinach Soup (page 216)

SNACK: Lentil–Quinoa Burger (page 205)

DESSERT: Chocolate Pumpkin Pudding (page 231)

Summer Meal Plan

DAY ONE

MEAL ONE: Peanut Butter Smoothie (page 235)

MEAL TWO: Raw Watermelon and Tomato Salad (page 212)

MEAL THREE: Zucchini Pasta with Tomato Sauce (page 219)

SNACK: Almond Milk and Apricot Muesli (page 221)

DAY TWO

MEAL ONE: Strawberry–Oatmeal Smoothie (page 240)

MEAL TWO: Portobello Mushroom Burger and Chopped Salad with Dijon Dressing (page 208 and page 198)

MEAL THREE: Citrus Gazpacho (page 199)

SNACK: Pineapple Almond Poppers (page 236)

DAY THREE

MEAL ONE: Quinoa with Fruit and Nuts (page 238)

MEAL TWO: Squash–Sunflower Seed Soup (page 214)

MEAL THREE: Black Bean Bowl (page 194)

SNACK: Chickpea–Red Pepper Salad (page 197)

DESSERT: Chocolate Ice Cream (page 230)

Shopping List: Staple Foods to Have on Hand

Whether you make a few recipes in this book from time to time or follow the meal plans diligently each season, having staples on hand will take a lot of the guesswork and hassle out of cooking. If you have the basics, you can whip up a meal in no time.

For the non-perishable items, purchase in bulk whenever possible. Since most recipes suggest just a tablespoon of nut butter here and there, I suggest simply having jars of nut butter on hand so you can make recipes without running out of products. Refer to the guide on how to store produce (page 182) so you get the most for your money.

SPICES AND OILS

Black pepper

Cayenne

Chili powder

Chili powder mix (often contains cumin, paprika, onion, etc. Look for salt-free brands.)

Cinnamon

Coconut oil

Coriander

Cumin

Dried onion flakes

Ground ginger

Nutmeg

Olive oil

Oregano

Paprika

BAKING INGREDIENTS

Baking powder

Baking soda

Honey or agave nectar

Spelt flour, buckwheat flour, or oat flour

Sucanat, coconut palm sugar, or date sugar

Vanilla extract (look for an alcohol-free variety if you have a gluten sensitivity)

PRODUCE

Acorn squash

Apples

Avocados

Bananas

Basil

Blueberries

Bok choy

Broccoli

Carrots

Cauliflower

Celery

Chiles

Chives

Cilantro

Cucumbers

Garlic

Garlic chives

Ginger

Grapefruit

Jalapeño peppers

Kale

Leeks

Lemons

Limes

Mesclun greens

Onions

Oregano

Parsley

Portobello mushrooms

Red cabbage

Red leaf lettuce

Red bell peppers

Red potatoes

Romaine lettuce

Scallions

Shiitake mushrooms

Spinach

Strawberries

Summer squash

Sweet potatoes

Tomatoes

Watermelon

White button mushrooms

Zucchini

DRIED FRUIT

Apricots

Cherries

Cranberries

Currants

Dates

Pineapple

Raisins

GRAINS AND LEGUMES

Black beans

Chickpeas

Lentils

Oats

Quinoa

Red beans

Sprouted brown rice

Sprouted brown rice tortillas

Sprouted gluten-free bread,
such as Manna Bread

Sprouted grain tortillas

NUTS AND SEEDS

Almonds

Cashews

Chia seeds

Flax seeds

Hemp seeds

Macadamia nuts

Pistachios

Pumpkin seeds

Sacha inchi seeds

Walnuts

NUT BUTTERS AND MILKS

Almond butter

Almond milk

Cashew butter

Coconut milk (found in the
ethnic/international foods aisle)

Hemp seed butter

Peanut butter

Sunflower seed butter

Tahini

SOY PRODUCTS

Though there are no soy products in the recipes, if you do eat soy, these are some of the best sources and can help boost health and protein intake. There is differing information on soy, so pay attention to how your body responds, as organic, non-GMO soy can be a wonderful source of complete protein and calcium.

Soybeans
Soy milk
Soy yogurt
Sprouted tofu
Tempeh

OTHER

Apple cider vinegar
Balsamic vinegar
Bragg's Liquid Aminos
Brown rice vinegar
Canned pure pumpkin
Cocoa and/or cacao powder
Coconut liquid aminos
Daiya Wedges or Shreds, Mozzarella or Cheddar
Dark chocolate or vegan chocolate
Dijon mustard
Frozen blueberries
Frozen strawberries
Hemp, pea, or brown rice protein powder
Low-sodium tomato juice
Low-sodium vegetable broth
Nutritional yeast
Quinoa or brown rice elbow macaroni pasta
Spirulina
Tomato paste

QUICKEST WAY TO SAVE MONEY AND EAT FOOD WITH A TON OF FLAVOR: PURCHASE WHAT'S IN SEASON.

CHAPTER 15

Power Vegan Tools

"Happiness is nothing more than good health and a bad memory."
—*ALBERT SCHWEITZER*

With plant-based living, as with any new way of life, sometimes it's good to get more than one opinion before you dive in. Whether you want to learn more about vegan living, eating raw, alkaline foods, or raising a child with a plant-based diet, check out the array of books, websites, and appliances that I have found helpful and that can make your job in the kitchen (and in life) much easier. Remember, as with anything new, it takes time to learn what's right for your body. Just because it's written doesn't mean it's right. *Always* follow your instincts about eating for your body and about feeding your family quality foods.

RESOURCES

Books
Baby Greens by Michaela Lynn and Michael Chrisemer, NC
Conscious Eating by Gabriel Cousens, MD
Dining in the Raw by Rita Romano
Eat Smart, Eat Raw by Kate Wood
Eat to Live by Joel Fuhrman, MD
Eating Animals by Jonathan Safran Foer
Eating for Beauty by David Wolfe
Enzyme Nutrition by Dr. Edward Howell
Everyday Raw by Matthew Kenney
Evie's Kitchen by Shazzie
Feasting on Raw Foods by Charles Gerras

Forks Over Knives edited by Gene Stone

Going Raw by Judita Wignall

Living on Live Food by Alissa Cohen

No More Dirty Looks by Siobhan O'Connor and Alexandra Spunt

Rainbow Green Live-Food Cuisine by Gabriel Cousens, MD

Raw: The Uncook Book by Juliano Brotman and Erika Lenkert

Raw Family by Victoria Boutenko, Igor Boutenko, Sergei Boutenko, and
   Valya Boutenko

Skinny Bitch by Rory Freedman and Kim Barnouin

Smoothies: 50 Recipes for High-Energy Refreshment by Sara Corpening
   Whiteford, Lori Lyn Narlock, and Mary Corpening Barber

Super Juice by Michael Van Straten

The Acid-Alkaline Diet for Optimum Health by Christopher Vasey

The Big Book of Juices and Smoothies by Natalie Savona

The Children's Health Food Book by Ron Seaborn

The China Study by T. Colin Campbell and Thomas M. Campbell II

The Complete Book of Raw Food edited by Julie Rodwell

The Complete Idiot's Guide to Plant-Based Nutrition by Julieanna Hever, MS,
   RD, CRT

The Engine 2 Diet by Rip Esselstyn

The Happy Herbivore Cookbook by Lindsay S. Nixon

The Kind Diet by Alicia Silverstone

The Raw 50 by Carol Alt

The Raw Food Detox Diet by Natalia Rose

The Raw Gourmet by Nomi Shannon

The Raw Life by Paul Nison

The Vegan Sourcebook by Joanne Stepaniak

The Vegetarian 5-Ingredient Gourmet by Nava Atlas

Thrive by Brendan Brazier

Thrive Foods by Brendan Brazier

1,000 Vegan Recipes by Robin Robertson

Vegan for Life by Jack Norris, RD and Virginia Messina, MPH, RD

Vegan Nutrition: Pure and Simple by Michael Klaper, MD

Vegan on the Cheap by Robin Robertson

Warming Up to Living Foods by Elysa Markowitz

Why Suffer? By Ann Wigmore

Websites

Born to Love (natural products for infants and children): http://www.borntolove.com

Cherrybrook Kitchen (allergen-free products): http://www.cherrybrookkitchen.com

Choosing Raw: http://www.choosingraw.com

Crazy Sexy Life: http://www.crazysexylife.com

Door to Door Organics: http://www.doortodoororganics.com

Go Veg: http://features.peta.org/VegetarianStarterKit/

Gourmet Greens: http://www.gourmetgreens.com

Happy Cow: http://www.happycow.net

Hip Mama: http://www.hipmama.com

Living Right: http://livingrightfoods.com/

LoveToKnow Vegetarian: http://vegetarian.lovetoknow.com

Meatless Monday: http://www.meatlessmonday.com

Organic Athlete: http://www.organicathlete.org

Peapod (grocery delivery): http://www.peapod.com

Sunfood: http://www.sunfood.com

Super Vegan: http://supervegan.com

T. Colin Campbell Foundation: http://www.tcolincampbell.org

The China Study Community: http://www.thechinastudy.com

Veg News: http://vegnews.com

Vega: http://www.myvega.com

Vegan.com: http://vegan.com

Vegan Bodybuilding & Fitness: http://www.veganbodybuilding.com

Vegan Outreach: http://www.veganoutreach.org

Whole Foods Market: http://www.wholefoodsmarket.com

YumUniverse: http://www.yumuniverse.com

Films

Chow Down

Fat, Sick & Nearly Dead

Food Fight

Food, Inc.

Food Matters

Forks Over Knives

King Corn

Our Daily Bread

Simply Raw: Reversing Diabetes in 30 Days

Super Size Me

Sweet Misery: A Poisoned World

The Future of Food

The Price of Sugar

Vegucated

KITCHEN TOOLS

Blenders

Good: Oster 6-Cup Glass Jar 7-Speed Blender

Better: Blendtec Total Blender

Best: Vitamix CIA Professional Series

Cutting Boards

Good: MIU Flexible Cutting Boards

Better: Architec The Gripper Bamboo Cutting Board

Best: Ironwood Gourmet Acacia Wood Large End Grain Prep Station

Dehydrators

Good: Waring DHR30 Professional Dehydrator

Better: L'Equip 306200 500-Watt 6-Tray Food Dehydrator

Best: Excalibur 3900 Deluxe Series 9-Tray Food Dehydrator

Food Processors

Good: Cuisinart Pro-Classic 7-Cup Food Processor

Better: KitchenAid 9-Cup Food Processor with 4-Cup Mini Bowl

Best: Breville Sous Chef Food Processor

Juicers

Good: Hamilton Beach Big Mouth Juice Extractor

Better: Breville Juice Fountain Compact, 700-Watt

Best: Omega Nutrition Center Commercial Masticating Juicer

Knives

Good: J.A. Henckels Five Star 8-inch Chef's Knife

Better: Wüsthof Classic 9-inch Chef's Knife

Best: Global 8-inch Chef's Knife

Mixing Bowls

Good: Pyrex 3-Piece Mixing Bowl Set

Better: Trudeau Plastic Bowl Set

Best: All-Clad Stainless Steel Mixing Bowls

APPENDIX

Arsenal of Power Vegan Exercises

In this section, I've included descriptions of all the exercises mentioned in Chapters 10 and 11. I have also demonstrated some of the more complicated exercises with step-by-step photos. These photos are included to assist you with the proper form (disclaimer: They were taken five months post pregnancy, so be kind).

Many of the following exercises use a "row" and/or a "clean" movement. Here are some definitions:

- **Row:** This term means to lift a weight by pulling the arms in toward the body, flexing the muscles of the back, and bending your elbows to complete the movement. (See photos of Barbell Swim, page 256.)
- **Clean:** Using your trapezius muscles (the flat triangular muscles of your shoulder and upper back), shrug the weights up to your shoulders as you drop into a squat. Flip your wrists up toward the ceiling to "catch" the weights by your shoulders. This should be a fast and powerful movement. (See photos of Clean and Press, page 261.)

BARBELL SWIM: Grasp a light barbell in front of you at shoulder height with both hands. Bend right elbow back and straighten left arm. Move fluidly to bending the other elbow, "rowing" arms as if you were swimming. Keep the barbell at shoulder height throughout the movement.

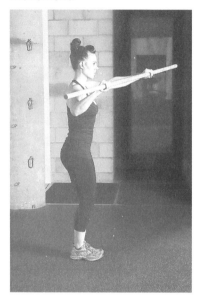 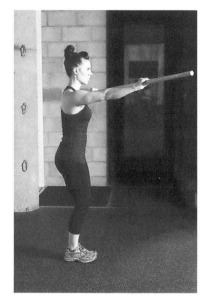

Barbell Swim

BEAR CRAWL: Begin on hands and knees. Knees should be bent, hands directly under shoulders. Begin to crawl forward by bending your left knee and moving it forward (your left knee should almost kick your left elbow). Keep your butt down and continue moving forward with your right arm and leg. Alternate arms and legs crawling forward, using your core to propel you forward. Try not to swivel your hips.

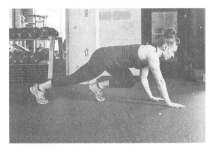 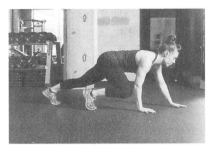

Bear Crawl

BOX JUMP: Begin by facing a low/medium step or bench. Squat slightly, keeping your back flat and core engaged. Spring up, landing with both feet firmly on top of the bench in a semi-squat or deep squat. Hop or step back down.

BRIDGE: Lie down on a mat and bend your knees, feet flat on the floor. Try to move your heels close to your butt. Slide hands down the length of your back toward your heels, and clasp hands together underneath your lower back as you lift your hips and bottom off the ground. Tighten the backs of your legs as you lift hips higher. Try to pinch shoulder blades together. Hold for 10–30 seconds. Come down. Repeat three times.

BROAD JUMP: Find an open space. Squat, swinging your arms back. Propel your body forward and land softly on your heels, sinking into a squat. Continue jumping forward for all reps.

BROAD JUMP TO WALK-OUT PUSH-UP WITH BEAR CRAWL BACK:
Perform a Broad Jump. Immediately walk hands out to push-up position. Perform a Walk-Out Push-Up and walk hands back to standing.
Continue moving forward with Broad Jumps and Walk-Out Push-Ups
for reps. Then perform a Bear Crawl moving backwards to the start.

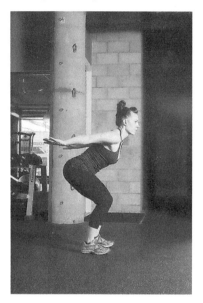
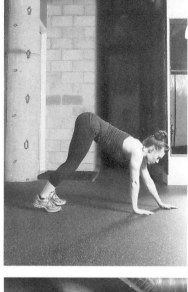

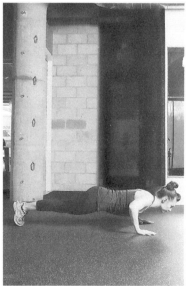
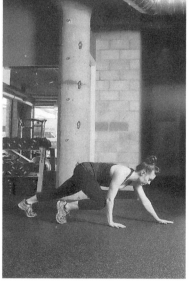

Broad Jump to Walk-Out Push-Up with Bear Crawl Back

BRONCO BURPEE: Squat and place hands on the floor. Using your core, shoot both legs up to the ceiling into a handstand. Lower both legs back down and jump straight up in the air. Repeat for all reps.

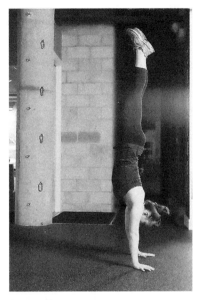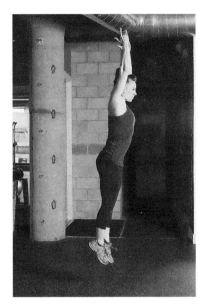

Bronco Burpee

BURPEE: Squat until your hands are touching the floor. Shoot your feet back to a push-up position, hop them back in to your hands, and stand up, jumping up at the top.

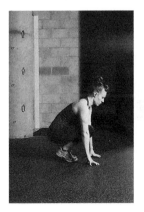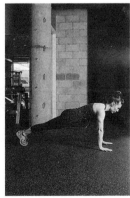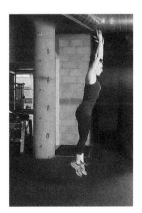

Burpee

CABLE TWIST: Face a cable that is positioned at about hip height. Load it up with a medium weight. Grasping one handle in both hands with an overhand grip, use your abs to slice the cable over to your right hip, back to center, then over to the left.

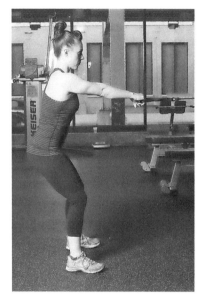 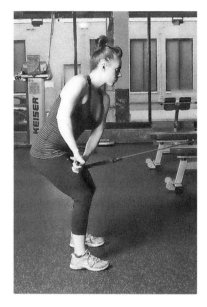

Cable Twist

CHEST TAP PUSH-UP: Begin in push-up position. Perform a push-up and spring from bent elbows into the air, tapping the chest and then lowering back into a push-up.

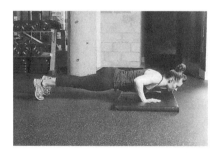 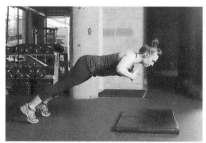

Chest Tap Push-Up

CLEAN AND PRESS: Hold a barbell in front of your body, palms down. Using your shoulders and core, "clean" the barbell up to your shoulders by rowing up, and then bend your elbows forward and flip your wrists so the barbell is at your clavicles. Press barbell up overhead, stopping before elbows are locked. Return to start.

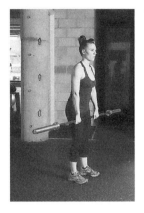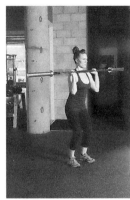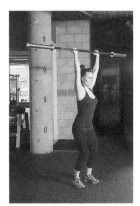

Clean and Press

CLEAN AND PRESS FROM KNEES: Begin on your knees, a barbell in front of you. Keeping your back flat, hop to your feet and quickly perform a Hang Clean (see page 266). Press weight overhead. Return barbell to the ground and hop back to knees.

DEADLIFT: Place a barbell on the ground in front of you and grasp it with both hands, palms facing down or with an alternating grip. Keeping a flat back and sinking into a deep squat, lift the barbell until you are standing and lean back slightly, squeezing your hamstrings. Try to sit back and use your hamstrings to lower the weight to the ground. Repeat for all reps.

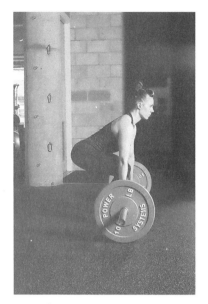 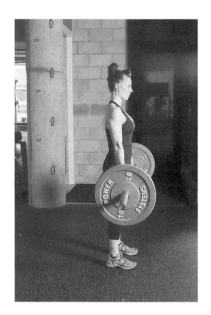

Deadlift

DEADLIFT FROM KNEES: Begin on knees with barbell in front of you. Hop to feet and perform a **deadlift**, keeping a flat back. Lower to start and repeat.

DECLINE SPIDER PLANK: Find a low bench. Get in front of it in a push-up position and prop your toes on the bench. Make sure your wrists are under your shoulders. Bend one knee, driving it out to the side and up toward your elbow. Pause, return to start, and repeat with other leg.

DROP SQUAT: Begin with feet shoulder-width apart. Drop quickly into a squat position and stand up. Immediately drop again, keeping a quick pace for all reps.

DOWNWARD-FACING DOG: Walk hands out to a push-up position and then push your hips up and back until your body is making an upside-down V. Try to press back into your heels. Keep your back flat and shoulders away from your ears. Take as many deep, cleansing breaths as possible.

FIGURE 8: Grasp a dumbbell, plate, kettle bell, or medicine ball with left hand. Lower into a semi-squat and feed the weight behind your legs with left hand, catching it with the right hand beside the right thigh. Bring weight up to shoulder height and feed through to the opposite side. Continue this smooth motion for all reps.

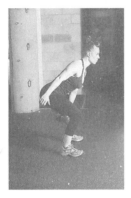 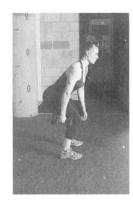 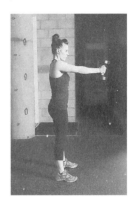

Figure 8

FULL BOSU SIT-UP: Begin with your back on a Bosu ball or cushioned mat. With fists balled in front of chin, knees bent, and feet firmly on the floor, crunch up and into a standing position, throwing two punches at the top. Slowly sit and lower body back onto the Bosu ball, extending back until abs are flat. Repeat.

FULL PARTNER TWISTING CRUNCH: Lie on your back, butt to butt with a partner, with your legs pointing straight into the air. Position both of your hips over to the left so that your hips are side by side. Grasp each other's hands out by your sides. Digging hands into mat, lift both of your tailbones, rotate tailbones to the right, and set hips down gently. Lift and rotate to left. You should be lifting up and over each other, using the core to complete each repetition.

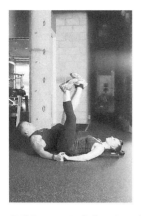 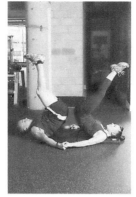 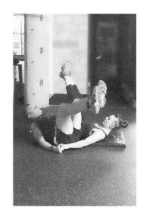

Full Partner Twisting Crunch

GET-UP: Begin standing, with your left side facing a wall. Extend left arm out and touch the wall. Keeping the left hand on the wall, sit down, bending left knee up and sliding right leg in front of left, with inside of right foot parallel to ceiling. Tap the bottom of the right foot against wall. Using your core, pop right foot back behind you and up to standing (imagine you are popping up on a surfboard). Complete reps on one side and repeat on the other.

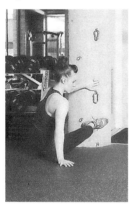 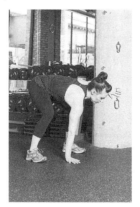 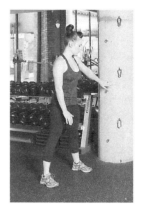

Get-Up

HALO: Grasp a heavy plate in front of your body. Using your core and shoulders, lift the plate in front of your face, around toward your right ear, and behind your head, making a circle. Once the plate reaches the front of your body, bring it down to your right hip in a fluid motion. Pause and reverse movement to bring around left ear, behind head, and down to the left hip. Repeat.

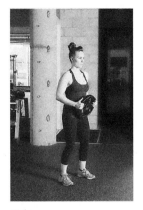 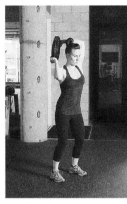 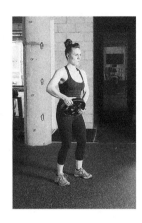

Halo

HANDSTAND: Stand in front of a wall or enlist the help of a friend. With your arms by your ears, step right foot forward as you place your hands on the ground, and let the left leg swing up behind you and into a handstand. Bring right leg to meet it. Hold. Kick back down slowly to start.

HANDSTAND PUSH-UP: Face a wall or sturdy surface. Raise arms next to ears and place right foot in front of left. Kick left leg up and back as you push off right leg to bring yourself into a handstand against the wall. Once stable, bend elbows into a vertical push-up. Pause, then straighten arms. Repeat for all reps before kicking down.

HANG CLEAN: Hold a barbell in front of your body, palms down. Using your shoulders and core, "clean" the barbell up to your shoulders by rowing up, and then bend your elbows forward and flip your wrists so the barbell is at your clavicles. Lower to start, and repeat.

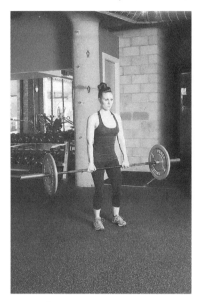 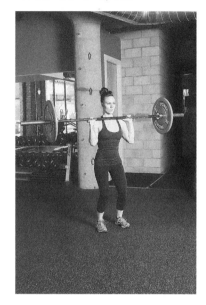

Hang Clean

HANG CLEAN FROM KNEES: Begin on your knees, a barbell in front of you. Keeping your back flat, hop to your feet and quickly perform a hang clean. Lower barbell to ground and return to knees.

HANG CLEAN INTO REVERSE LUNGE: Perform a hang clean and, once the barbell is at chest height, step left foot back and lower into a lunge. Return to start. Perform another hang clean and, at the top, lower into a lunge with the opposite leg.

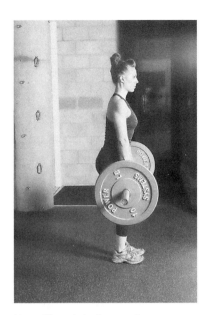
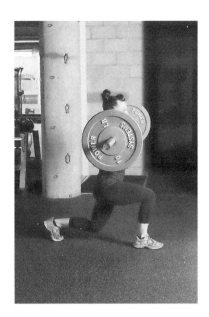

Hang Clean into Reverse Lunge

HIP ESCAPE: Start in push-up position. Lifting your right hand, shoot your left leg through toward the right, keeping it in line with your hip. You should be resting the outside of your left foot on the ground and should almost be sitting down on your left butt cheek. Keep your right leg bent, knee up, toes pointing back. Quickly bring that leg back through and to push-up position and then, seamlessly, lift left hand and shoot right leg through. This is one rep. Continue this smooth motion, focusing on your core for all reps.

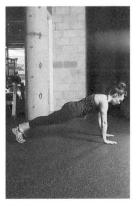
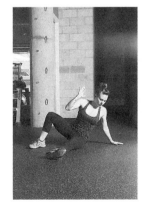
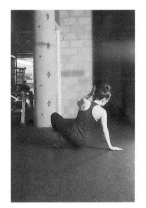

Hip Escape

INCHWORM: Stand tall and place hands on the ground in front of you. Walk hands out to push-up position, and immediately walk feet in to meet hands. Walk hands out again to push-up position and walk feet in. Complete for all reps.

INCLINE PUSH-UP: Face a bench. Place hands on bench, wider than chest-width apart, and walk feet back and adjust until body is in one straight line (push-up position). Engage core and make sure back is flat. Perform a push-up, only lowering until chest is even with bench. Push through chest and return to start. Repeat for all reps.

KAMIKAZE PUSH-UP: Bend knees and touch hands to floor in front of you. You should be in a crouched position. Explode back into a push-up, then jump up to a crouched position. Repeat.

KNEES: Wear a mitt on your dominant hand, stacking the other hand on top of it. Face your palms downward. Step left foot in front of right. Drive right knee into the mitt, leaning back from hips, and keeping mitt at hip height. Step right foot back behind left and step left foot back to meet right. Step right foot in front of left and then drive left knee up into mitt. Step left foot back to meet right and continue alternating for reps.

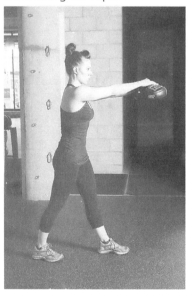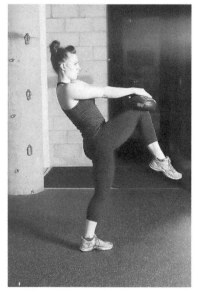

Knees

LATERAL HOP: Stand with feet together. Lower into a semi-squat and then hop to the right, letting the left foot land behind the right. Immediately spring back to the left, crossing right foot behind left. Repeat for all reps.

LATERAL SHUFFLE: Bend knees. With a flat back, shuffle a few paces to the right, keeping hips facing front. Shuffle back to the left.

LATERAL SHUFFLE WITH BURPEE: Bend knees and shuffle two paces to the right. Drop into a Burpee. Jump up and shuffle two paces to the left. Drop into a Burpee. Repeat for all reps.

MAN-MAKER: Holding medium weights, get into a push-up position. Perform a push-up and, at the top of the push-up, row one of the weights up to your side. Perform another push-up and row the other weight up to your other side. Shoot both feet in toward your hands and, using your core, "clean" the weights up to your shoulders as you drop into a squat and stand. Press them overhead. Return to start. This is one rep.

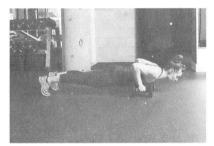
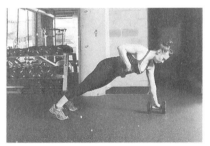

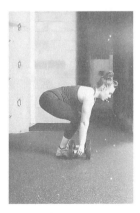
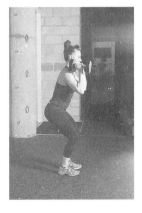
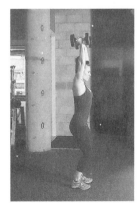

Man-Maker

MEDICINE BALL SPRAWL: Place a medium medicine ball on the ground and, with both hands still on it, jump your feet back wider than hip-width. Press hips towards the ground. Using your core, hop feet back in and lift the ball back to chest height. This is one rep.

MEDICINE BALL TWIST: You will need to have a sturdy wall or partner for this one. Begin on your knees on a mat, holding a medicine ball. Your left shoulder should be facing a wall. Toss the ball towards the wall, twisting from your core. Catch it and twist to the right. Then twist back to the left to toss ball back against the wall. Complete for reps and then switch to other side.

MOUNTAIN CLIMBER: Begin on hands and toes. Tighten core and drive right knee up to chest, then switch. Continue in a quick motion, tapping toes lightly on the floor as you switch. (You can also make this harder by driving knees to opposite shoulders.)

PLANK JACK: Begin in a plank position, either on elbows and toes or hands and toes. Keeping your hips still, jump the legs out slightly wider than hips and then back in, concentrating on keeping your core tight and your back nice and straight. Keep jumping legs in and out for reps.

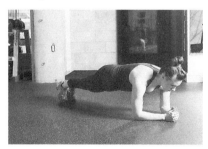 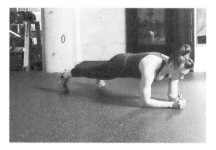

Plank Jack

PLANK MOGUL: Begin on hands and toes. Bend knees and jump feet in and up by your right shoulder. Return to start. Jump feet in and up toward your left shoulder. Continue alternating, using the core to complete each movement.

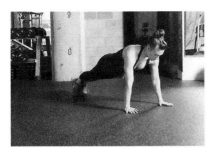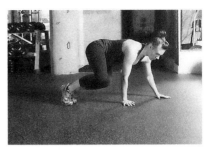

Plank Mogul

PLATE DRAG: Begin on your hands and toes with a plate under your feet. Bend your knees and drag the plate in towards your chest. Immediately walk the hands out to push-up position. Bring the legs in and walk the hands out. Repeat.

PLATE PUSH: Set a heavy plate on a carpet or towel. Place hands on either side of it. Using your legs, drive the plate across an open space as far as you can. Keep core engaged. Push back to start to complete one set.

PRISONER JUMP SQUAT: Place hands behind head. Lower into a squat. Before returning, push off of legs to jump up and land softly in a squat. Repeat.

PRISONER SQUAT: Place hands behind head. Lower body into a squat, keeping knees stable and behind toes. Sit like you are sitting in a chair. Return to standing.

PULL-UP: Find a high, stable bar and stand below it. Hang with a wide overhand grip and use your back to pull yourself up to the bar. Control the movement on the way down. Repeat.

PULL-UP TO BURPEE: Stand in front of a stable high bar. Jump into a wide-grip Pull-Up. Lower slowly and hop back down to the ground. Immediately squat, place hands on the ground, and shoot legs back into push-up position. Perform one push-up. Hop feet back in and jump back into a Pull-Up. Repeat.

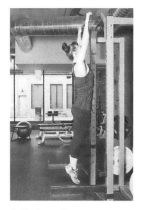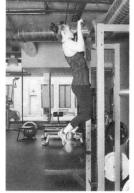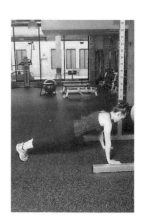

Pull-Up to Burpee

PUNCH: Grab two medium dumbbells and hold them in front of your chin, elbows in, shoulders relaxed. Place one foot in front of the other. Bend your knees. Tightening your core, extend left arm out, rotating dumbbell to face the floor. Retract left arm and extend right arm. Rotate from the core for all punches.

RENEGADE ROW: Grab two medium dumbbells and get into push-up position. Without moving hips, row one weight up to your ribs, using your back. Lower to ground and repeat with other weight.

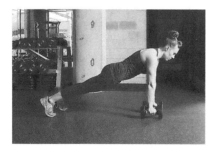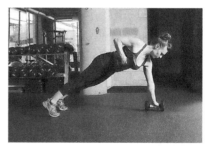

Renegade Row

RESISTED KNEES: Loop a resistance-band handle around a low, steady surface. Place the other handle on top of your left foot. With a mitt on your dominant hand, step your right foot in front of your left. Drive left knee into mitt, leaning back slightly. Repeat for all reps and then switch sides.

RESISTED KNEES WITH SPRAWL: Loop a resistance-band handle around a low, steady surface. Place the other handle on top of your left foot. Wear a mitt on your dominant hand. Step right foot in front of left until you feel some resistance. Drive left knee up into mitt and step back. Immediately shoot feet back into plank (or wider, into a sprawl with hips pressing into the ground), and stand. Repeat all reps on one side and then switch.

REVERSE BURPEE: Squat and place hands on the ground. Shoot legs back into push-up position. Immediately walk hands in to meet feet and shoot feet back into a push-up position again. Continue for reps.

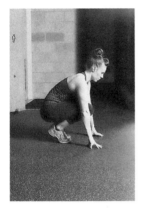 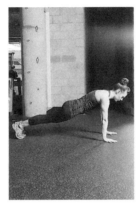 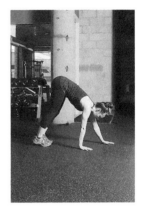

Reverse Burpee

REVERSE CRUNCH: Lie on your back. Place both hands under your tailbone or by your sides. Lift hips up, straighten legs, and act as though you are stamping your feet on the ceiling. Use only the core for this movement. Repeat for all reps.

SCARECROW: Hold two medium dumbbells in front of your body, palms facing body. Perform an upright row by pulling the weights up toward your chin, keeping your elbows high (you should look like a scarecrow). At the top, rotate elbows back until weights are at shoulder height. Rotate back to upright row and lower to start. Repeat.

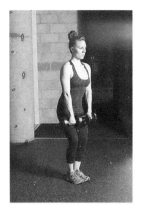
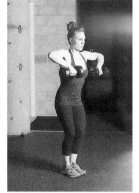
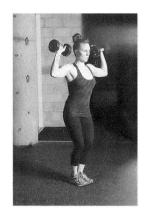

Scarecrow

SHOULDER STAND: Lie on your back on a mat, arms by your sides. Lift your hips off the floor and bring your legs up, over, and beyond your head. Move your hands toward your back and, if you can, place your hands on the small of your back. Straighten your spine and lift your lower body into the air to make one straight line with your hips and legs. Gently hold pose and ease out of it back to start.

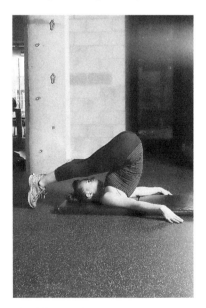
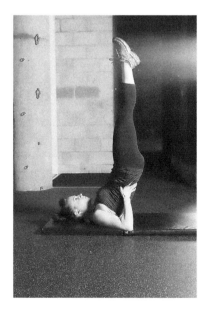

Shoulder Stand

SHOULDER THROW: Standing in front of a cable machine (or attaching a resistance band to a steady surface), attach a handle to a low cable. Grab it with both hands. Stand with left foot in front of right and extend arms straight in front of you. Twisting your torso and legs, "throw" the cable over to your left shoulder, bending your legs. Return to start. Repeat for all reps and switch sides.

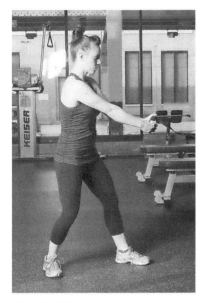 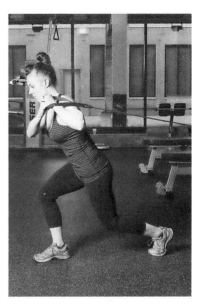

Shoulder Throw

SINGLE-ARM BARBELL CHEST PRESS: Lie on your back on a flat bench or incline bench, legs separated and feet on floor. With one hand, grasp a medium barbell directly in the middle. Find your balance and then slowly bend elbow to 90 degrees, using the chest to lower the weight. Pause at chest height and return to start. Complete reps and then switch sides.

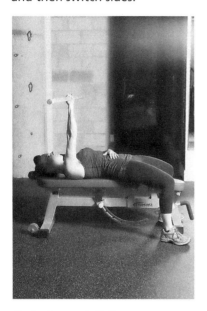 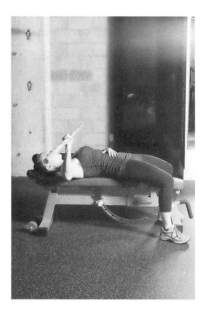

Single-Arm Barbell Chest Press

SINGLE-LEG BURPEE: Begin with feet together, standing tall. Lift left leg slightly off floor. Squat down, place hands on the floor, and shoot right leg back into a plank, keeping left leg close to right. Shoot right leg back in to a squat and hop up to standing. Hop on that same foot at the top, lifting arms overhead. Return to Burpee. Complete all reps and then switch sides.

SINGLE-LEG DEADLIFT: Begin standing, legs together, holding a weight in your left hand. Lift your left leg slightly behind you and hinge forward from the hips, keeping your back flat and letting left leg extend completely behind you. Lower the weight toward the ground near right foot, keeping hips square to the front. Squeeze the back of your right leg. Return to start and sweep your left leg through and to the front of your right leg. Immediately sweep it behind and lower into another rep. Perform all reps on one side before switching sides.

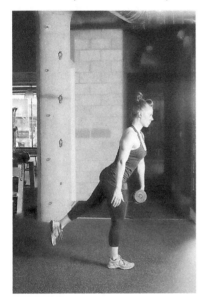 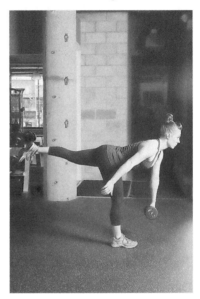

Single-Leg Deadlift

SINGLE-LEG DEADLIFT TO HOP: Begin standing with legs together. Lift your left leg slightly behind you and hinge forward from the hips, keeping your back flat. Lower left hand toward the ground near right foot, keeping hips square to the front. Squeeze the back of your right leg. Return to start and sweep your left leg through. Bend left knee and push off your right foot to hop straight up in air. Land and lower back to deadlift. Repeat for all reps and then switch sides.

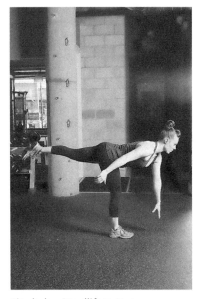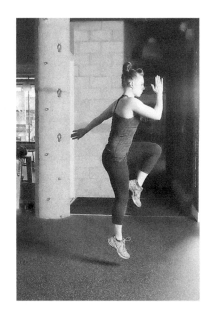

Single-leg Deadlift to Hop

SLAP PUSH-UP: Begin in a push-up position, facing a partner or a wall. Perform a push-up. At the top, extend right arm out and tap your partner's right hand, or the wall. Perform another push-up and tap the left hand. Repeat.

SMITH MACHINE PULL-UP: Set bar to thigh height. Grab bar and walk body beneath it until you are in one straight line. Extend arms straight, then bend, pulling chest up to meet the bar. Return to start.

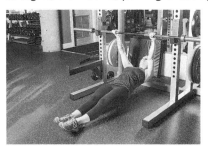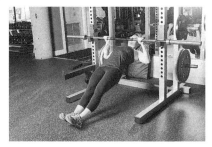

Smith Machine Pull-Up

SPIDER PLANK: Begin in a push-up position on your hands and toes. Lift your right leg, bending the knee out to the side, like you are trying to kick yourself in the elbow. Use the core, instead of the momentum from your leg, to perform this movement. Return to start and repeat with other leg.

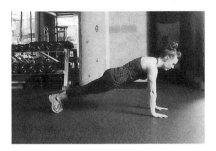 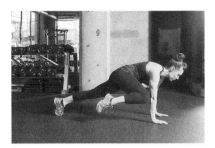

Spider Plank

SPRINT: Whether outside or on a treadmill, opt for 4 to 6 20-second sprints during your workout. Make sure you are warmed up and then sprint as hard as you can for the allotted time. Increase the intensity by starting from a knee or both knees, or from your stomach.

SQUAT WITH ONE-ARM TWISTING ROW: Grasp a medium dumbbell in right hand. Squat, letting the weight hang between legs. Return to standing and immediately row the dumbbell up and to the right, twisting your torso to the right. The elbow should be the highest point of the movement. Lower back to start. Repeat for all reps and then switch sides.

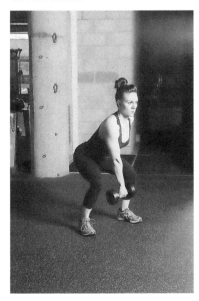 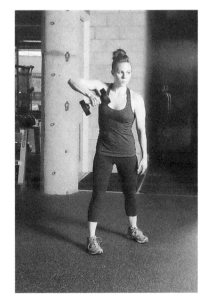

Squat with One-Arm Twisting Row

STEP-UP INTO REVERSE LUNGE: Begin with feet together, hands on hips, facing a step or bench. Step onto the bench with your right leg, bringing your left knee up to hip height. Contract your core. Step down with the left leg and immediately lower right leg behind left into a reverse lunge (see image of Hang Clean into Reverse Lunge, on page 267). Complete all reps with right leg before switching sides.

THUMBS UP: Begin on hands and toes in a push-up position. Without swiveling hips, extend right arm with thumb up into the air directly in front of shoulder. Switch arms and repeat.

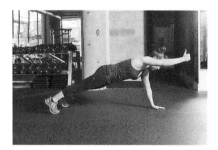 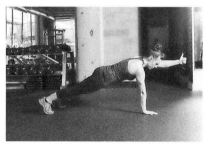

Thumbs Up

TOWEL ROW: Drape a towel over a low bar or Smith Machine set to around thigh height. Grab the ends of the towel and walk body out until you are under the bar, legs extended, body in one straight line. Pull your body up to the bar, using your back and core. Return to start.

TWISTING REVERSE CRUNCH: Lie on your back, legs straight up in the air, hands out to your sides. Lifting your tailbone off the ground, act like you are stamping your feet on the ceiling. At the same time you lift, twist your hips, so you are making a corkscrew with your lower body. Lower back to start and repeat on other side, twisting to the other side. This is one rep.

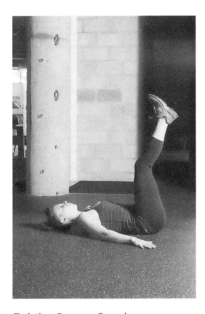 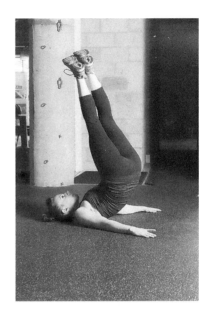

Twisting Reverse Crunch

WALK-OUT PUSH-UP: Begin by standing tall, feet together. Place hands on floor in front of you and walk hands out to push-up position. Lower into a push-up. Walk hands back to start and stand. Repeat.

NOTES

Chapter 1

[1] Veronique L. Roger, MD, MPH, FAHA, Alan S. Go, MD, Donald M. Lloyd-Jones, MD, ScM, FAHA, Emilia J. Benjamin, MD, ScM, FAHA, Jarett D. Berry, MD, William B. Borden, MD, Dawn M. Bravata, MD et al., on behalf of the American Heart Association Statistics Committee and Stroke Statistics Subcommittee, "Heart Disease and Stroke Statistics—2012 Update: A Report from the American Heart Association," *Circulation* 125 (2012): e2–e220, doi: 10.1161/CIR.0b013e31823ac046.

[2] "Noncommunicable Diseases (NCD)," World Health Organization Global Health Observatory, http://www.who.int/gho/ncd/en/index.html.

[3] Michael F. Picco, M.D., "Digestion: How Long Does It Take?," Mayo Clinic, http://www.mayo-clinic.com/health/digestive-system/an00896.

[4] Centers for Disease Control and Prevention, "National Diabetes Fact Sheet: National Estimates and General Information on Diabetes and Prediabetes in the United States, 2011" (Atlanta, GA: US Department of Health and Human Services, Centers for Disease Control and Prevention, 2011).

Chapter 2

[5] Joshua Rosenthal, *Integrative Nutrition: Feed Your Hunger for Health & Happiness* (New York: Integrative Nutrition, 2008), 62.

[6] Rosenthal, *Integrative Nutrition*, 63.

[7] Lynn, Michaela, and Michael Chrisemer, NC, *Baby Greens: A Live-Food Approach for Children of All Ages* (Berkeley: Frog Books, 2004), 9.

[8] Lynn and Chrisemer, *Baby Greens*, 9-10.

[9] Lynn and Chrisemer, *Baby Greens*, xvii.

Chapter 3

[10] Justin McCurry, "Japan's Centenarian Population Reaches More than 50,000," *The Guardian*, September 14, 2012, http://www.guardian.co.uk/world/2012/sep/14/japan-centenarian-population.

[11] Colin T. Campbell and Thomas M. Campbell II, *The China Study: The Most Comprehensive Study of Nutrition Ever Conducted and the Startling Implications for Diet, Weight Loss, and Long-Term Health* (Dallas: BenBella Books, 2006), 6.

[12] Rory Freedman and Kim Barnouin, *Skinny Bitch Bun in the Oven: A Gutsy Guide to Becoming One Hot and Healthy Mother!* (Philadelphia: Running Press, 2008), 89.

[13] Food and Agricultural Organization of the United Nations, *Livestock's Long Shadow* (Rome: Food and Agricultural Organization of the United Nations, 2006), http://www.fao.org/docrep/010/a0701e/a0701e00.htm.

[14] Lynn and Chrisemer, *Baby Greens*, 21.

[15] Physicians Committee for Responsible Medicine, "Health Concerns About Dairy Products," http://www.pcrm.org/health/diets/vegdiets/health-concerns-about-dairy-products.

Chapter 4

[16]John Robbins, "The Truth About Calcium and Osteoporosis," http://foodmatters.tv/articles-1/the-truth-about-calcium-and-osteoporosis.

[17]Gabriel Cousens, MD, *Conscious Eating,* as quoted in Freedman and Barnouin, *Skinny Bitch Bun in the Oven,* 69.

[18]Cousens, *Conscious Eating,* as quoted in Freedman and Barnouin, *Skinny Bitch Bun in the Oven,* 71–78.

Chapter 5

[19]Rosenthal, *Integrative Nutrition,* 142.

[20]Joel Fuhrman, *Eat to Live: The Amazing Nutrient-Rich Program for Fast and Sustained Weight Loss* (New York: Little, Brown, 2003), 21.

[21]Furhman, *Eat to Live,* 21-22; G.S. Berenson, S.R. Srinivasan, W. Bao, et al., "Association Between Multiple Cardiovascular Risk Factors and Atherosclerosis in Children and Young Adults: The Bogalusa Heart Study," New England Journal of Medicine 338, no. 23 (June 4, 1998): 1650–56.

[22]Berenson, Srinivasan, Bao, et al., "The Bogalusa Heart Study," as quoted in Furhman, *Eat to Live,* 21–22.

Chapter 6

[23]Kimberly Snyder, "Studies Show Peanuts May be Hazardous To Your Health," October 25, 2012, http://kimberlysnyder.net/blog/2012/10/25/peanuts-health-food-or-hazardous-to-your.health.

[24]Stephanie Bailey, "Bug Food: Edible Insects," University of Kentucky College of Agriculture, Entomology Department, http://www.ca.uky.edu/entomology/dept/bugfood1.asp; US Food and Drug Administration, "Defect Levels Handbook: The Food Defect Action Levels," last updated November 9, 2011, http://www.fda.gov/food/guidancecomplianceregulatoryinformation/guidancedocuments/sanitation/ucm056174.htm.

Chapter 8

[25]Brazier, Brendan. *Thrive: The Vegan Nutrition Guide to Optimal Performance in Sports and Life* (Philadelphia: Da Capo, 2007), 125.

[26]Joseph Mercola. "Finally People Starting to Consume Less Sugar!" Food Consumer, August 16, 2011, http://www.foodconsumer.org/newsite/mobile/Nutrition/Food/sugar_0816111141.html.

Chapter 9

[27]Brazier, *Thrive,* 127.

Chapter 11

[28]John Robbins, *Diet for a New America,* as quoted in Freedman and Barnouin, *Skinny Bitch Bun in the Oven,* 68.

[29]Siobhan O'Connor and Alexandra Spunt, *No More Dirty Looks: The Truth about Your Beauty Products—and the Ultimate Guide to Safe and Clean Cosmetics* (New York: Da Capo, 2010), 70; Ruth Winter, *A Consumer's Dictionary of Cosmetic Ingredients,* 5th ed. (New York: Three Rivers Press, 1999), 455.

Chapter 12

[30]Rosenthal, *Integrative Nutrition,* 120.

[31]"Spoiled Rotten—How to Store Fruits and Vegetables," *Vegetarian Times,* 2013, http://www.vegetariantimes.com/article/spoiled-rotten-how-to-store-fruits-and-vegetables.

[32]"Spoiled Rotten—How to Store Fruits and Vegetables," *Vegetarian Times.*

[33]"Spoiled Rotten—How to Store Fruits and Vegetables," *Vegetarian Times.*

REFERENCES

Alt, Carol. *The Raw 50: 10 Amazing Breakfasts, Lunches, Dinners, Snacks, and Drinks for Your Raw Food Lifestyle.* New York: Clarkson Potter, 2007.

Brazier, Brendan. *Thrive: The Vegan Nutrition Guide to Optimal Performance in Sports and Life.* Philadelphia: Da Capo, 2007.

————. *Thrive Foods: 200 Plant-Based Recipes for Peak Health.* Cambridge, MA: Da Capo, 2011.

Campbell, T. Colin, and Thomas M. Campbell II. *The China Study: The Most Comprehensive Study of Nutrition Ever Conducted and the Startling Implications for Diet, Weight Loss, and Long-Term Health.* Dallas: BenBella Books, 2006.

Davis, Brenda, RD, and Vesanto Melina, MS, RD. *Becoming Vegan: The Complete Guide to Adopting a Healthy Plant-Based Diet.* Summertown, TN: Book Publishing Company, 2000.

Lynn, Michaela, and Michael Chrisemer, NC. *Baby Greens: A Live-Food Approach for Children of All Ages.* Berkeley: Frog Books, 2004.

Foer, Jonathan Safran. *Eating Animals.* New York: Little, Brown, 2009.

Fuhrman, Joel. *Eat to Live: The Amazing Nutrient-Rich Program for Fast and Sustained Weight Loss.* New York: Little, Brown, 2003.

Freedman, Rory, and Kim Barnouin. *Skinny Bitch Bun in the Oven: A Gutsy Guide to Becoming One Hot and Healthy Mother!* Philadelphia: Running Press, 2008.

Norris, Jack, RD, and Virginia Messina, MPH, RD. *Vegan for Life: Everything You Need to Know to Be Healthy and Fit on a Plant-Based Diet.* Boston: Da Capo, 2011.

O'Connor, Siobhan, and Alexandra Spunt. *No More Dirty Looks: The Truth about Your Beauty Products—and the Ultimate Guide to Safe and Clean Cosmetics.* New York: Da Capo, 2010.

Rosenthal, Joshua. *Integrative Nutrition: Feed Your Hunger for Health & Happiness.* New York: Integrative Nutrition, 2008.

INDEX

ABOUT THE AUTHOR

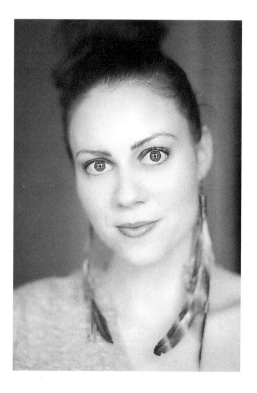

Rea Frey is an author, nutrition specialist, and International Sports Sciences Association certified trainer. She has done extensive research on plant-based diets and overall nutrition and has been a practicing plant eater for the last 15 years. She is the author of *The Cheat Sheet: A Clue-by-Clue Guide to Finding Out if He's Unfaithful* (Adams Media, June 2011) and has been featured in *Fitness, Ladies' Home Journal,* and *Whole Living.* She lives in Chicago and blogs about her workout routines, recipes, and life as a vegan mom at www.reafrey.com. (And yes, those earrings in her photo are cruelty free.)